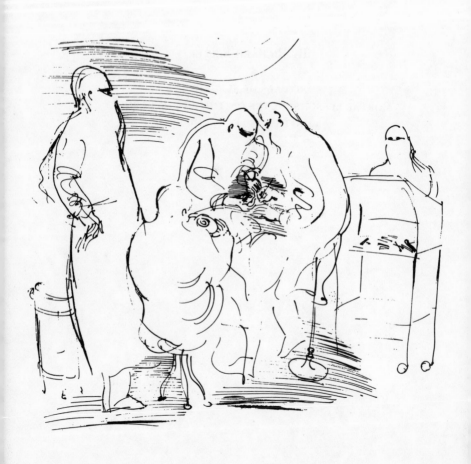

RICHARD SELZER

CONFESSIONS OF A KNIFE

A Touchstone Book
Published by Simon and Schuster
New York

First Touchstone Edition, 1981
Published by Simon and Schuster
A Division of Gulf & Western Corporation
Simon & Schuster Building
Rockefeller Center
1230 Avenue of the Americas
New York, New York 10020

TOUCHSTONE and colophon are trademarks of Simon & Schuster

Designed by Eve Metz

Manufactured in the United States of America

1 2 3 4 5 6 7 8 9 10

1 2 3 4 5 6 7 8 9 10 Pbk.

Library of Congress Cataloging in Publication Data

Selzer, Richard.

Confessions of a Knife.

1. Selzer, Richard. 2. Surgeons—United States—
Biography. 3. Surgery—Anecdotes, Facetiae, Satire,
etc. 1. Title.
RD27.35.S44A33 617'.092'4 [B] 79-12670
ISBN 0-671-24292-X
ISBN 0-671-41385-6 Pbk.

Parts of this book originally appeared in *New England Review, Antaeus, Harper's, Esquire, Connecticut Magazine* and *Mademoiselle.*

The author wishes to thank Macmillan, Inc., for permission to reprint two lines from "The Wild Old Wicked Man" by W.B. Yeats, copyright 1940 by Georgie Yeats, renewed 1968 by Bertha Georgie Yeats, Michael Butler Yeats, and Anne Yeats.

ACKNOWLEDGMENTS

I would like to express my thanks to Yaddo where much of this book was written. My gratitude extends as well to Nan Talese for her sensitive editing, to Chris Hatchell for his imaginative and technical assistance, and to Enid Rhodes Peschel for her inspired criticism.

TO MY MOTHER, GERTRUDE

CONTENTS

I

II

III

Illustrations

The Operation, *Raoul Dufy.*   4
Musée Municipal d'Art Moderne, Paris.

L'Accident, *Auguste Leper (after a lithograph by*   13
Pascal Adolphe Jean Dagnau-Bouveret. Yale Medical
Library.

Crippled Beggar, *Jacques Callot.*   61
Bibliothèque Nationale, Paris.

Anatomical Plate, *Charles Bell.*   157
Library of the Medical Faculty, University of Paris.

I

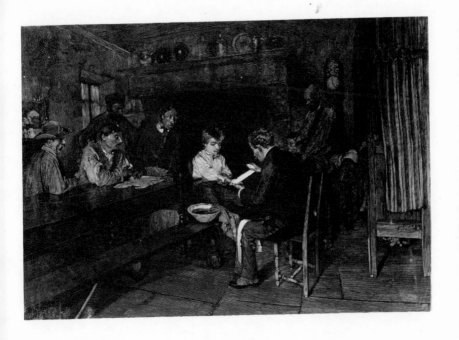

AN ABSENCE OF WINDOWS

NOT LONG AGO, operating rooms had windows. It was a boon and a blessing in spite of the occasional fly that managed to strain through the screens and threaten our very sterility. For the adventurous insect drawn to such a ravishing spectacle, a quick swat and, Presto! The door to the next world sprang open. But for us who battled on, there was the benediction of the sky, the applause and reproach of thunder. A Divine consultation crackled in on the lightning! And at night, in Emergency, there was the pomp, the longevity of the stars to deflate a surgeon's ego. It did no patient a disservice to have Heaven looking over his doctor's shoulder. I very much fear that, having bricked up our windows, we have lost more than the breeze; we have severed a celestial connection.

Part of my surgical training was spent in a rural hospital in eastern Connecticut. The building was situated on the slope of a modest hill. Behind it, cows grazed in a pasture. The operating theater occupied the fourth, the ultimate floor, wherefrom huge windows looked down upon the scene. To glance up from our work and see the lovely cattle about theirs, calmed the frenzy of the most temperamental of prima donnas. Intuition tells me that our patients had fewer wound infections and made speedier recoveries than those operated upon in the airless sealed boxes where now we strive. Certainly the surgeons were of a gentler stripe.

I have spent too much time in these windowless rooms. Some part of me would avoid them if I could. Still, even here, in these bloody closets, sparks fly up from the dry husks of the human body. Most go unnoticed, burn out in an instant. But now and then, they coalesce into a fire which is an inflammation of the mind of him who watches.

Not in large cities is it likely to happen, but in towns the size of ours, that an undertaker will come to preside over the funeral of a close friend; a policeman will capture a burglar only to find that the miscreant is the uncle of his brother's wife. Say that a fire breaks out. The fire truck rushes to the scene; it proves to be the very house where one of the firemen was born, and the luckless man is now called on to complete, axe and hose, the destruction of his natal place. Hardly a civic landmark, you say, but for him who gulped first air within those walls, it is a hard destiny. So it is with a hospital, which is itself a community. Its citizens—orderlies, maids, nurses, x-ray technicians, doctors, a hundred others.

A man whom I knew has died. He was the hospital mailman. It was I that presided over his death. A week ago I performed an exploratory operation upon him for acute surgical abdomen. That is the name given to an illness that is unknown, and for which there is no time to make a diagnosis with tests of the blood and urine, x-rays. I saw him writhing in pain, rolling from side to side, his knees drawn up, his breaths coming in short little draughts. The belly I lay the flat of my hand upon was hot to the touch. The slightest pressure of my fingers caused him to cry out—a great primitive howl of vowel and diphthong. This kind of pain owns no consonants. Only later, when the pain settles in, long and solid, only then does it grow a spine to sharpen the glottals and dentals a man can grip with his teeth, his throat. Fiercely then, to hide it from his wife, his children, for the pain shames him.

In the emergency room, fluid is given into the mailman's veins. Bags of blood are sent for, and poured in. Oxygen is piped into his nostrils, and a plastic tube is let down into his stomach. This, for suction. A dark tarry yield slides into a jar on the wall. In another moment, a second tube has sprouted from his penis, carrying away his urine. Such is the costume of acute surgical abdomen. In an hour, I know that nothing has helped him. At his wrist, a mouse skitters, stops, then darts away. His slaty lips insist upon still more oxygen. His blood pressure, they say, is falling. I place the earpieces of my stethoscope, this ever-asking Y, in my ears. Always, I am comforted a bit by this ungainly little hose. It is my oldest, my dearest friend. More, it is my lucky charm. I place the disc upon the tense mounding blue-tinted belly, gently, so as not to shock the viscera into commotion (those vowels!), and I listen for a long time. I hear nothing. The bowel sleeps. It plays possum in the presence of the catastrophe that engulfs it. We must go to the operating room. There must be an exploration. I tell this to the mailman. Narcotized, he nods and takes my fingers in his own, pressing. Thus has he given me all of his trust.

A woman speaks to me.

"Do your best for him, Doctor. Please."

My best? An anger rises toward her for the charge she has given. Still, I cover her hand with mine.

"Yes," I say, "my best."

An underground tunnel separates the buildings of our hospital. I accompany the stretcher that carries the mail-man through that tunnel, cursing for the thousandth time the demonic architect that placed the emergency room in one building, and the operating room in the other.

Each tiny ridge in the cement floor is a rut from which rise and echo still more vowels of pain, new sounds that I have never heard before. Pain invents its own language. With this tongue, we others are not conversant. Never mind, we shall know it in our time.

We lift the mailman from the stretcher to the operating table. The anesthetist is ready with still another tube.

"Go to sleep, Pete," I say into his ear, my lips so close it is almost a kiss. "When you wake up, it will all be over, all behind you."

I should not have spoken his name aloud! No good will come of it. The syllable has peeled from me something, a skin that I need. In a minute, the chest of the mailman is studded with electrodes. From his mouth a snorkel leads to tanks of gas. Each of these tanks is painted a different color. One is bright green. That is for oxygen. They group behind the anesthetist, hissing. I have never come to this place without seeing that dreadful headless choir of gas tanks.

Now red paint tracks across the bulging flanks of the mailman. It is a harbinger of the blood to come.

"May we go ahead?" I ask the anesthetist.

"Yes," he says. And I pull the scalpel across the framed skin, skirting the navel. There are arteries and veins to be clamped, cut, tied, and cauterized, fat and fascia to divide. The details of work engage a man, hold his terror at bay. Beneath us now, the peritoneum. A slit, and we are in. Hot fluid spouts through the small opening I have made. It is gray, with flecks of black. Pancreatitis! We all speak the word at once. We have seen it many times before. It is an old enemy. I open the peritoneum its full length. My fingers swim into the purse of the belly, against the tide of the issuing fluid. The pancreas is swollen, necrotic; a dead fish that has gotten tossed in, and now lies spoiling across the upper abdomen. I withdraw my hand.

"Feel," I invite the others. They do, and murmur against the disease. But they do not say anything that I have not heard many times. Unlike the mailman, who was rendered eloquent in its presence, we others are reduced to the commonplace at the touch of such stuff.

We suction away the fluid that has escaped from the sick pancreas. It is rich in enzymes. If these enzymes remain free in the abdomen, they will digest the tissues there, the other organs. It is the pancreas alone that can contain them safely. This mailman and his pancreas—careful neighbors for fifty-two years until the night the one turned rampant and set fire to the house of the other. The digestion of tissues has already begun. Soap has formed here and there, from the compounding of the liberated calcium and the fat. It would be good to place a tube (still another tube) into the common bile duct, to siphon away the bile that is a stimulant to the pancreas. At least that. We try, but we cannot even see the approach to that duct, so swollen is the pancreas about it. And so we mop and suck and scour the floors and walls of this ruined place. Even as we do, the gutters run with new streams of the fluid. We lay in rubber drains and lead them to the outside. It is all that is left to us to do.

"Zero chromic on a Lukens," I say, and the nurse hands me the suture for closure.

I must not say too much at the operating table. There are new medical students here. I must take care what sparks I let fly toward such inflammable matter.

The mailman awakens in the recovery room. I speak his magic name once more.

"Pete." Again, "Pete," I call.

He sees me, gropes for my hand.

"What happens now?" he asks me.

"In a day or two, the pain will let up," I say. "You will get better."

"Was there any . . . ?"

"No," I say, knowing. "There was no cancer. You are clean as a whistle."

"Thank God," he whispers, and then, "Thank *you*, Doctor."

It took him a week to die in fever and pallor and pain.

It is the morning of the autopsy. It has been scheduled for eleven o'clock. Together, the students and I return from our coffee. I walk slowly. I do not want to arrive until the postmortem examination is well under way. It is twenty minutes past eleven when we enter the morgue. I pick the mailman out at once from the others. Damn! They have not even started. Anger swells in me, at being forced to face the *whole* patient again.

It isn't fair! Dismantled, he would at least be at some remove . . . a tube of flesh. But look! There is an aftertaste of life in him. In his fallen mouth a single canine tooth, perfectly embedded, gleams, a badge of better days.

The pathologist is a young resident who was once a student of mine. A tall lanky fellow with a bushy red beard. He wears the green pajamas of his trade. He pulls on rubber gloves, and turns to greet me.

"I've been waiting for you," he smiles. "Now we can start."

He steps to the table and picks up the large knife with which he will lay open the body from neck to pubis. All at once, he pauses, and, reaching with his left hand, he closes the lids of the mailman's eyes. When he removes his hand, one lid comes unstuck and slowly rises. Once more, he reaches up to press it down. This time it stays. The gesture stuns me. My heart is pounding, my head trembling. I think that the students are watching me. Perhaps my own heart has become visible, beating beneath this white laboratory coat.

The pathologist raises his knife.

"Wait," I say. "Do you always do that? Close the eyes?"

He is embarrassed. He smiles faintly. His face is beautiful, soft.

"No," he says, and shakes his head. "But just then, I remembered that he brought the mail each morning . . . how his blue eyes used to twinkle."

Now he lifts the knife, and, like a vandal looting a gallery, carves open the body.

To work in windowless rooms is to live in a jungle where you cannot see the sky. Because there is no sky to see, there is no grand vision of God. Instead, there are the numberless fragmented spirits that lurk behind leaves, beneath streams. The one is no better than the other, no worse. Still, a man is entitled to the temple of his preference. Mine lies out on a prairie, wondering up at Heaven. Or in a many windowed operating room where, just outside the panes of glass, cows graze, and the stars shine down upon my carpentry.

TILLIM

THE BOY'S FACE is the color of the Torah, as though in the years of bending over the scrolls, his skin had become infiltrated with something, a vapor, that rose from the parchment. But here inscribed with acne. He seems almost another species, a thin messy breed, with a nose too large for the narrow recessed mandible below. Metal bands all but hide his yellow teeth. A blue velvet yarmulke pinned to his dark hair is embroidered in heavy gold thread. From beneath his shirt hang the four fringes of a prayer shawl. They are dirty, glutinous. He plays with them, twisting the threads in his fingers. It is private, automatic.

"How old are you?" I ask him.

"Seventeen."

He looks to be thirteen or fourteen. The strangeness, the unkemptness distance me. I am very tired.

"What is the matter?"

"I have an ingrown toenail," he says. "It is infected."

"Climb up on the table," I say. He does so, not sitting on the edge and bracing his hands to lift himself, but facing the table, putting up first one knee, then the other, kneeling there, hesitating, and finally turning to a sitting position. The roll of paper covering the table tears. It has taken him a full minute to do this.

"Take off your shoe." It is the end of the day. I am growing snappish. He does.

"Your sock, please."

The left big toe is swollen and red. Pus has gathered there where the nail is deeply embedded in the flesh. Part of the nail will have to be cut away.

"Lie down, please." Each time, he complies, but only just. He uses his whole body to delay. I force my voice to gentleness.

"You will feel two needle pricks, one at either side at the base of the toe. Not in the sore part." I show him where.

All at once, he sits up. He is agitated. He cannot control his terror.

"After that," I say, "you will feel nothing. Your toe will be numb."

In a loud voice and with an edge of desperation, he calls out to his father who is in the waiting room.

"Tateh! Tateh!"

A man opens the door of the examining room. He is tall and handsome, with a red beard and blue, German eyes. He is wearing an impeccable new fedora. One finger keeps his place among the pages of a black leather-bound book. The barest tips of spotless white fringes show beneath his jacket.

"Shah! Shah!" He speaks firmly, coldly to the boy. His face is taut with anger. The presence of the man calms, domesticates the boy.

"Lie down, please," I say to the boy. I wipe his toe with alcohol on a sponge, and advance with the syringe. But he draws back his foot, twists free. There is no violence in him. He cannot do it. He just *cannot*.

All right then, I think. Don't give in. There has already been too much submission. But I am tired.

"Let's get this over with," I say.

"Why don't you call upon your spiritual resources?" I say. It is a mean remark. I am ashamed of having said it. But somehow, it is a suggestion that he can accept. He lies still upon the table, covers his eyes with one arm, and lets come from his lips an unceasing silken whisper of Hebrew. I grasp the toe firmly with one hand, pinching it and bending it down. Not out of callousness. It is to distract him from the prick of the needle. Still, there is pain. The whisper pauses, but only for an instant, then rushes on. The first injection has been given.

"What is it that you are reciting?" I ask him.

The whisper has stopped, but he does not answer.

"*Tillim*," says the father. "Hebrew psalms."

"That is a good thing to do," I say. "Here is the last needle."

Again the whisper, and I am made sorrowful by the sound. He seems far away from me, exalted. I think of the others who went to the sealed chambers murmuring *tillim*. I think of this ancient sibilance mingling with the hiss of gas.

"Now there will be no more pain," I say. Firmly, I massage the base of the toe to hasten the spread of the anesthetic in the tissues. I insert one blade of the scissors beneath the toenail and advance toward the base, cutting until the root of the nail is divided.

"Where do you go to school?"

"I go to the yeshiva. In New York," he says. He is animated.

"I come home for weekends. There is very strict discipline there." He smiles. "With boys," he says, "you need discipline." He looks at his father and smiles faintly. I know from his voice that he needs none. He has never done any rebellious thing. He cannot.

I grasp that third of the toenail that is to be removed, with a heavy clamp. With a sharp tug, I avulse it from the nail bed. It comes away intact.

"Do you have brothers?"

"No. I am the only one. That is why I have trouble getting along with the other boys."

I turn to the father. "Are you a rabbi?"

"No."

"What do you do?"

"I am a businessman." He looks down, smooths the crease of his pants.

"But still I study Talmud," he says. "Every day."

With a scalpel, I cut away the overgrown infected tissue. Then I cauterize it with silver nitrate. I bandage the toe. Only when he is certain that the toe is concealed by the dressing, only then does the boy raise his head to look down. Abruptly, he sits up. His agitation returns, but it is different. It is not fear that goads him, but something no less intense, as though he were pursuing an idea, a knowledge, ferreting it out. It is a truth that he *must* know. He needs it. In order to survive after his body has been put to torture, some piece of it slain. The questions pour from him. Exactly what did you do? How should I take care of it? Will it be all right from now on? Are you sure it will not come back? Will it hurt when the anesthetic wears off? He asks the same things over and over. It is a kind of talmudic questioning.

"Can I see your scissors?" he asks. I hand them to him. His blood still wets the blades.

"Oh," he says, "my blood!" And he draws in his breath. He wears the handle of the scissors on his thumb and forefinger, and snips at the air. This movement, too, is awkward. His fingers are tangled. He opens the scissors to their widest, and reads aloud.

"Made in Germany." He falls silent. I think that he will ask no more questions. But he does. "Can I see it?" he asks.

"Can you see what?"

"My toenail. The part you cut off."

I pick up the fragment of the toenail with a forceps, and deposit it on a gauze sponge.

"Here," I say, and hold up the sponge for him to see.

Ignoring the gauze, he takes up the nail in his fingers. He holds it close to his face, studying it. So close . . . for a moment I am afraid that he is going to pop it into his mouth. Suddenly, with a swift movement, he throws the toenail on the floor.

"Ach," he says and wipes his hand on his fringe. "Feh!" He shudders, and smiles faintly.

I should make him pick it up, I think. But I do not.

Later, when they have gone, I bend to pick up the toenail. I hold it in my palm for a little time, then lift it to the light. It is translucent. At the margins, where it is reddened with the boy's blood, there is a glow, as of stained glass. At last, I go to flick the nail into the trash can. But it sticks to my fingers. It will not leave me. In the end, I grasp it with the steel forceps and tap the instrument against the rim of the can. The toenail falls then, and, as the lid drops shut, there is a blazing–up within the receptacle as though something has been ignited.

FOUR APPOINTMENTS
WITH THE DISCUS THROWER

ONE

I SPY on my patients. Ought not a doctor to observe his patients by any means and from any stance, that he might the more fully assemble the evidence? So I stand in the doorways of hospital rooms and gaze. Oh, it is not all that furtive an act. Those in bed need only look up in order to discover me. But they never do.

From the doorway of Room 542, the man in the bed seems deeply tanned. Blue eyes and close-cropped white hair give him the appearance of vigor and good health. But I know that his skin in not brown from the sun. It is rusted, rather, in the last stage of containing the vile repose within. And the blue eyes are frosted, looking inward like the windows of a snowbound cottage. This man is blind. This man is also legless—the right leg missing from midthigh down, the left from just below the knee. It gives him the look of an ornamental tree, roots and branches pruned to the purpose that the thing should suggest a great tree but be the dwarfed facsimile thereof.

Propped on pillows, he cups his right thigh in both hands. Now and then, he shakes his head as though acknowledging the intensity of his suffering. In all of this, he makes no sound. Is he mute as well as blind?

If he is in pain, why do I not see it in his face? Why is the mouth not opened for shrieking? The eyes not spun skyward? Where are tears? He appears to be waiting for something, something that a blind man cannot watch for, but for which he is no less alert. He is listening.

The room in which he dwells is empty of all possessions —the get-well cards, the small private caches of food, the day-old flowers, the slippers—all the usual kickshaws of the sickroom. There is only a bed, a chair, a nightstand, and a tray on wheels that can be swung across his lap for meals. It is a wild island upon which he has been cast. It is Room 542.

TWO

"What time is it?" he asks.

"Three o'clock."

"Morning or afternoon?"

"Afternoon."

He is silent. There is nothing else he wants to know. Only that another block of time has passed.

"How are you?" I say.

"Who is it?" he asks.

"It's the doctor. How do you feel?"

He does not answer right away.

"Feel?" he says.

"I hope you feel better," I say.

I press the button at the side of the bed.

"Down you go," I say.

"Yes, down," he says.

He falls back upon the bed awkwardly. His stumps, un-weighted by legs and feet, rise in the air, presenting them-selves. I unwrap the bandages from the stumps, and begin to cut away the black scabs and the dead glazed fat with scissors and forceps. A shard of white bone comes loose. I pick it away. I wash the wounds with disinfectant and redress the stumps. All this while, he does not speak. What is he thinking behind those lids that do not blink? Is he remembering the burry prickle of love? A time when he was whole? Does he dream of feet? Of when his body was not a rotting log?

He lies solid and inert. In spite of everything, he remains beautiful, as though he were a sailor standing athwart a slanting deck.

"Anything more I can do for you?" I ask.

For a long moment he is silent.

"Yes," he says at last and without the least irony, "you can bring me a pair of shoes."

In the corridor, the head nurse is waiting for me.

"We have to do something about him," she says. "Every morning he orders scrambled eggs for breakfast, and instead of eating them, he picks up the plate and throws it against the wall."

"Throws his plate?"

"Nasty. That's what he is. No wonder his family doesn't come to visit. They probably can't stand him any more than we can."

She is waiting for me to do something.

"Well?"

"We'll see," I say.

THREE

The next morning, I am waiting in the corridor when the kitchen delivers his breakfast. I watch the aide place the tray on the stand and swing it across his lap. She presses the button to raise the head of the bed. Then she leaves.

In this time, which he has somehow identified as morning, the man reaches to find the rim of the tray, then on to find the dome of the covered dish. He lifts off the cover and places it on the stand. He fingers across the plate until he probes the eggs. He lifts the plate in both of his hands, sets it on the palm of his right hand, centers it, balances it. He hefts it up and down slightly, getting the feel of it. Abruptly, he draws back his right arm as far as he can.

There is the crack of the plate breaking against the wall at the foot of his bed and the small wet sound of the scrambled eggs dropping to the floor. Just so does this man break his fast.

And then he laughs. It is a sound you have never heard. It is something new under the sun.

Out in the corridor the eyes of the head nurse narrow.

"Laughed, did he?"

She writes something down on her clipboard.

A second aide arrives, brings a second breakfast tray, puts it on the nightstand out of his reach. She looks over at me, shaking her head and making her mouth go. I see that we are to be accomplices.

"I've got to feed you," she says to the man.

"Oh, no you don't," the man says.

"Oh, yes I do," the aide says, "after what you just did. Nurse says so."

"Get me my shoes," the man says.

"Here's oatmeal," the aide says. "Open." And she touches the spoon to his lower lip.

"I ordered scrambled eggs," says the man.

"That's right," the aide says.

I step forward.

"Is there anything I can do?" I say.

"Who are you?" the man asks.

FOUR

In the evening, I go once more to that ward to make my rounds. The head nurse reports to me that Room 542 is deceased. She has discovered this quite by accident, she says. No, there had been no sound. Nothing. It's a blessing, she says.

I go into his room, a spy looking for secrets. He is still there in his bed. His face is relaxed, grave, dignified, as the faces of the newly dead are. After a while, I turn to leave. My gaze sweeps the wall at the foot of the bed, and I see the place where it has been repeatedly washed, where the wall looks very clean and very white in contrast to the rest, which is dirty and gray.

RACCOON

"DON'T COME IN! Stay out!"

Just so does the woman answer my knocking. But I am already inside the room. On hospital rounds, a knock is only a gesture.

"Are you all right?" I ask her through the bathroom door. There is no answer.

"I'll be back in a few minutes. Please get back in bed. I want to examine you." I turn to leave. Then I see advancing from beneath the closed door the blot of dark shine. I step closer. I crouch, peering. I slide open the door which separates us. In a hospital the doors cannot be locked.

The woman is naked. She sits on the toilet, bent forward, her pale white feet floating on the jammy floor. Nearby, a razor blade dropped from one painted hand. The other hand cannot be seen; it is sunk to the wrist within the incision in her abdomen. Bits of black silk, still knotted, bestrew the floor about her feet. They are like the corpses of slain insects. The elbow which points out from her body moves in answer to those hidden fingers which are working . . . working.

For a moment she does not seem to notice that I am there. Her face is turned upward, its gaze fixed on some galaxy beyond me. It is vacant, ecstatic. Something has fled from it. What does she knead? For what is she reaching? A precious coin that she will, *must* deliver herself of? A baby? And so she dilates the opening with her fist, and so gropes for the limbs of her fetus?

For a moment I cannot move or speak. I have been struck and minted at that spot. But then she sees me. And her face leaps back across vast distances. Now she is a woman surprised at her most secret act.

"You should not have come in," she says. Her voice is gaunt, quiet. "I was almost finished. You should have waited."

Her hand remains immersed in her body. She does not withdraw it. But now the elbow is still.

"What are you doing!" I say. "What have you done! Stand up here and come back to bed!"

"I almost had it," she says.

"What? What did you 'almost have'? You have opened up your incision. It is only five days since your operation. That was a terrible thing to do. Stand up now," I say firmly. "Come with me."

Then, more gently: "It's all right. Don't worry. We'll fix it. You didn't realize . . ."

I take her by the arm, lifting, and as I do, the plunged hand is extracted with a small wet sound. It is a fist, shiny, beaded with yellow globules of fat.

But a fist is a mystery. I must see what it holds. I pry open the fingers, all bridged with clots. It is raw and scalded . . . and empty. She whimpers, but not in pain. It is longing that she expresses. She sighs, and stands. A sash of intestine hangs from her belly. I reach one hand to cup it, to keep it from prolapsing further. The loop shudders in my palm.

The woman lies on the bed. I call out for assistance. In a moment a nurse arrives.

"Oh!" says the nurse quietly, and sucks back her saliva.

"Get me gauze packing, Betadine solution, instruments, and gloves."

Gently, I replace the coil of intestine inside the abdominal cavity. I clamp and suture the few points that are still bleeding. I pack the wound with yards of gauze, and drench it with the Betadine.

"That would really be painful, wouldn't it?" the woman asks me. "If that were my real body, I mean. It would hurt. But I don't feel anything at all."

All at once I know what it was, what she was reaching for, deep inside. It was her pain! The hot nugget of her pain that, still hissing, she would cast away. I almost had it, she said. You should have waited, she said.

Like a raccoon, I think. A raccoon whose leg is caught in a trap. A raccoon will gnaw through his thigh, cracking the bone between his jaws, licking away the blood and the fur. So has she torn open her incision to rummage in the furnace of her body for the white ingot inside. I close my eyes and see the raccoon rise. He hobbles from the trap. He will not die *there*. Now he turns his beautiful head to glance back at his dead paw. His molten eyes are full of longing.

But this woman feels no pain at my probing, my packing. Perhaps she is wrong. Perhaps she did find what she was looking for, and threw it away. Perhaps I did wait long enough.

"When you are calm," I say, "we'll go back to the operating room, and I will stitch you up again."

"I *am* calm," she says. "You are the one who isn't calm."

34

AMAZONS

THERE ARE TEN ROOMS in the operating theater of the hospital where I work. They open five each into two corridors which are the limbs of a V. Between these rooms are small foyers containing deep-bellied sinks where we scrub our hands. Here is the sound of running water, the splash and chatter of people. It is the custom among surgeons to visit the operating rooms of other surgeons. So do we learn from one another, take strength from the sight of others doing our work, give encouragement. It is a way, too, of measuring ourselves, as athletes do who attend games as spectators.

I have finished one operation and am waiting to begin another. The room in which I am working must be cleaned and prepared. For this time, I have entered the room adjacent to mine to learn, to encourage, to measure. An operating room is not a quiet place. The voices of men rise and fall. Orders are given. There is anger. One hears laughter. Somewhere a machine bubbles. Electronic beeping counts out the rhythm of a heart, and always there is the to-and-fro sough of breathing that is controlled by a hand squeezing a rubber bag. But this operating room that I visit is quiet. There is none of the clangor that punctuates these labors. In this room, voices are used softly. They murmur.

They purr. The wrists of these surgeons are slender, their fingers fine. When men huddle about an operating table, their heads bowed between bulky shoulders, they have the appearance of strength and mass. They group, like buffalo. But these, in this room, are deer. Their necks are long. They turn them like deer. They are women.

I see that I am the only male in the room. The others, surgeons, assistants, anesthesiologist, and nurses, all are women. And the patient, too. The operation is called mastectomy.

The anesthesiologist whispers to the patient, soothing her.

"Now you will go to sleep," she says. "It is not unpleasant."

She croons as though to a child.

"Give in, and when you wake up, it will all be over. Good night."

This she says although it is early in the morning. The woman on the table smiles dreamily at the upside-down face of the woman standing at the head of the table, the one who is lulling her. Then the patient's gaze turns distant, sightless, shifts to the empty air, and dissolves. She is asleep.

The breasts of the patient are laid bare by one of the attendants. Gently, she unsnaps the cotton jacket from behind the neck of the sleeping woman, and slides it from her. Next, she folds the sheet neatly across the lower abdomen. The breasts of the woman are vulnerable. They are offered. A masked woman steps forward. She is wearing a cap and rubber gloves and the green cotton dress that is the uniform of this place. She takes up gauze squares, dips them in a cup of red liquid, and begins to paint the breasts of the woman on the table. The first splotch of red on her skin is shocking, an intimation. There is a pattern to her washing. Starting at the nipple of the right breast, she scrubs in circles that expand outward concentrically until the whole breast is colored. Over and over she does this, each time using a new gauze sponge. The armpit and the upper arm down to the elbow are scrubbed too, and the right half of the neck. Somehow, the woman knows when she has finished. She steps back from the table, and strips off her gloves.

Two other women have entered the room from the small antechamber. With the swinging door ajar, the sound of running water can be heard. They step toward the center of the room, their hands held up before them in a gesture fixed and ritual. Their arms are wet; water drips from their elbows. They are given towels, and dry their hands and arms with infinite care. The towels are taken from them, and the three women are dressed by the nurses in long gowns of the same green color. The gowns are tied at the back. Next, rubber gloves are held open for them, and they dive with their hands in a single quick movement. As waterbirds dive. Now they are dressed, and arrange themselves on either side of the table.

"Towels," says one of the women. She is given, one after the other, four towels which she lays about the breast of the woman on the table.

"Clips," she says, and with four clips she hooks the towels together.

"Drape," she says, and together the women cover the patient with large green linen sheets, all except for her right breast which presents through a rectangular hole in the drape. They are ready to begin.

Now, their voices drop so that, standing in a corner of the room, I can no longer hear their words, only a kind of choir, a blending. There are long silences. The women are fully engaged. They seem unaware of their surroundings, parts of a unified whole, just as colonies and cities comprise a great empire, or as the organs of a single body pulse within the same membrane. Flank to flank, they are pressed on either side of the table, parting only to join again as though deriving comfort from the touching, just as the beasts of a herd press, wary of a dispersal that is the way to danger and abandonment.

I do not step closer to the table to watch. Something holds me from it. I remain standing in the corner.

At last, one of the women steps back from the table, and I see, in the space she has left, the great red and yellow wound. I see that the breast is not there. She who stepped aside is cupping it aloft. An attendant holds up a cardboard container. She drops it in. I hear the moist, muffled sound it makes. The surgeon turns back to the table, and I can see the elbows of the women moving back and forth as they sew. Now and then a needle rises to the level of a shoulder and I catch sight of its gleam just before it plunges. They are fast and deft. In a few minutes it is done. They remind me of the wives of farmers I have watched as a boy, women expert at weeding, pruning, snapping off dead twigs, pinching away soiled leaves, and stepping with inadvertent grace between the dense vulnerable rows of the garden.

I peer between the standing women, and see the chest of the one who is supine. It is flat, closed with a row of black stitches, running up and down, where the breast had been. It is neat, solemn. The women apply a dressing to the incision. They step away from the table, peel off their gloves, and untie the drawstrings of each other's gowns at the back. It is sisterly. They lower their masks and smile at each other.

"Good job," they say. "Well done." And they massage their faces to wipe away the strain. They walk past me as they leave the room. They do not acknowledge that I am present. Perhaps they do not see me.

It is hours later, evening, and I am sitting in my study. Perhaps I fall asleep . . . perhaps I dream . . .

There is an island inhabited by fierce warrior women. In the middle of the island stands a great temple with marble steps and columns. A young woman is being led to an altar. She is bare to the waist. At the foot of the altar is a stone cauldron filled with fire; protruding from the flames, the handle of tongs. The girl lies upon the altar. A woman gives her wine to drink. Another woman scatters leaves from a basket upon the girl's breasts. There is chanting. A priestess steps forward. She grasps the right breast of the girl and elevates it. Another priestess withdraws the tongs from the cauldron, holds them aloft for a moment, then presses them to the chest of the girl, drawing them in a circle about the breast. This she does again and again, searing the flesh until the breast falls free into the hands of the other. There is no blood, only the smell of burning. All this while, the girl makes no sound. Nor does she move.

Unguents are smeared upon the wound by an attendant. The women dress the girl in a tunic that covers her remaining breast, and she is carried to a grove nearby. Everything here—bark, stones, boughs, even the squirrels—is touched by a golden light that is uncontaminated, healing. It is a light in which there can be no misunderstanding.

Now I see that all of them are thus—one-breasted. I understand that this must be so in order that they might the more easily draw the bow across the chest, unhampered by the breast. I understand. One must consider these things in the context of the times. Still, when I awaken, I am trembling. And I think of these priestesses, robed, entranced, anointed conduits for the speech of gods, stepping from behind curtained altars to do their awful rites. Where lived the men would dare domesticate these wild creatures?

And I think of these surgeons with their scalpels, hemostats, and sutures, and their bags and bags of blood. I imagine them at nightfall strumming the guitar, wearing rings, returning the glances of men. I think of how each day, just as I do, they touch the incandescent center of the human body. And whole notions of life dissolve into nothing. It is good.

IN THE SHADOW OF THE WINCH

IT IS THE GREAT vessels I am after. The aortic arch with its branches, the carotids, the subclavian. There is a man, you see, waiting at the hospital. His own aorta has blown. It is a thin-walled blister that crowds his chest, pressing upon his heart and lungs, eroding the high pile of his vertebrae. On one side, it is grooved by his ribs. Here and there, it is barnacled with plaques of calcium. At any moment, it will burst: when he sneezes, perhaps, or bends to tie his shoe. So I am here, harvesting the organs of beasts for transplantation.

A little money has been paid.

In my bag, a packet of sterile instruments, sterile jars, rubber gloves. Everything is ready.

This slaughterhouse is kosher. The Gentiles make the cut too low on the neck. We need as much length on the arteries as we can get. The slaughterer wears hip boots and a skullcap. He mutters prayers. Blessings, I imagine. He and I are joined here for different purposes. To the cattle it is all the same.

One is chosen. Compared to a cheetah or a python, she would be almost vegetable—slow, planted, something whose destiny it is to be bitten off and chewed, as she has mowed many meadows. Nor would I compare her to the performing hawk, whose grace is exteriorized to the interface that flames between wing and wind. No. A cow has none of the bestial graces. And in the shadow of the Winch, she falls clumsier still.

Commotion! Behind a gate too high for leaping, a wild eye backs away from the prod. There is a scudding, a sidewise bumping into walls.

There is the sound of chains, and another sound like bagpipes skirling. A great wheel turns. What a scrabbling of hoofs! The head of the cow dips, is no longer to be seen above the gate. Over a pulley set in the roof, the chain pulls taut. In a minute she is lifted, upside down, one hind leg grappled by the chain. First seen rising is that braceleted hoof. The hind leg follows, pulled rigid by the weight of the hoisted cow. The other hind leg is held out from the side. It is thick, like the thigh of a fat woman. After, come the rump and tail, the torso; then there is the head, eyes bursting, sweet blunt horns remonstrating.

Her passion begins. Only now, as she is assumed, does she begin to low. She extends her head to look about. Her moo stretches breath to the limit. Behind the gate, the others listen. They thump and shove, then fall still. I think they know.

The height is convenient for the man in the hip boots and skullcap. His knife flashes. He steps forward.

"Cut high," I say. "Last time, the carotids were too short."

The slaughterer is good. One stroke across the neck beneath the mandible. She is caught in mid-groan, her lips and tongue working on. The fall of her whole blood to the stone floor is like the plash of her endless urinations. For as long as it can, her heart pumps the steaming blood to the floor, to the drain at the center, where the flies wait. The rushing out of her blood causes her to turn and gyrate on the chain. Soon enough, the fall slows to a woven strand. It lazes. At last, a trickle, a wavy thread. Then, drop follows drop. And still, she revolves, graceful at last, floating, airborne, she who stumbled and twitched below.

Perhaps, had she not gone lovely, I would not reach up my hand to still her motion. But I do. My palm comes to rest upon her belly. I press, and the swinging stops. She hangs. Now it is that I feel transmitted to my touch, a stirring. It is muffled, fur covered. Yet it quickens, insists. Again! It kicks, soft, to knock at my mind. Who's there! What lingers here to complete itself!

A calf almost, almost lives, unmindful, seeing still a world enough and time, as only the fetal might. I step to face the belly of the cow, press my ear against the warm pink skin where the fine hairs whorl at the midline. Above, the velvety udders hang, touching my hair. There! I feel it again. It lives!

My knife! Hurry! I tear open the sterile pack and rummage for the knife. I have it! Now! One long slit, and I shall lift it free. My own blood hurtles. My lungs flood with it. I seem to be remembering my own birth, the battering choking abrading blinding of it, the loss of all that was moist and warm, the bright that was more than bright.

Now! I raise my knife.

But I do not cut into the belly of the cow. I pause; I think: there is pro; there is con. Human ruminations have ever been the ruination of cattle. My knife clatters to the floor.

But I am so close to the heat of the beast's underparts. Her smell! Once more I press my ear to her abdomen. As I do, yes, as I do, her forelegs take me gently about the hips, her hoofs dangling. It is a reflex, I know. I stand in the embrace, the delicate embrace of the creature that, beyond death, offers herself in place of her calf.

The winched cow has stopped her plink, plink dripping upon the stones.

The carcass roars with silence.

The winch unwinds. The meat is lowered.

43

AT SAINT RAPHAEL'S

Not long ago there were among the members of this hospital community a number of handicapped workers. These were often the victims of some long and terrible illness, or the survivors of repeated efforts to cure them. Or they were graduates of the psychiatric ward. Some had congenital defects: a vestigial arm, perhaps, with an epaulet of floppy fingers at the shoulder, or a harelip and cleft palate that had resisted reconstruction. Some were blind, others deaf. Here also, the massively obese and the unfattenably emaciated. I remember one nurse's aide, a great strong epileptic girl with a frizz of orange hair and the nose of a camel. Between seizures, Ida could outperform a whole battalion of her colleagues. Alas, her demons would rouse at the most inauspicious moments: during the retrieval of a bedpan from beneath a patient, say, or in the midst of one of her famous backrubs. To the unsuspecting patient in the bed, her bellowing, the wild fling of her spittle and the shuddering, as though to break her bones, was a sure sign that he had already passed into the flames of Moloch, and was now closeted forever among the Damned.

More gently afflicted was Joe Salvati, the iceman. It was before the days of those soulless machines that manufacture ice on each ward, and toward which one gives no single backward glance. Joe Salvati was a graduate of the orthopedic ward where generations of interns, residents, and their professors had endeavored to straighten his spine, even off his legs, and otherwise surgically redo a skeleton tipped and tilted in a marvelous profusion of angles and

44

planes. After a decade or two encased in a tonnage of plaster of paris, his body was studded with rivets, pins, and bars without any noticeable change in his configuration having been achieved. As though, in spite of everything, Joe insisted on being himself. He lurched and waggled as before, and the great hump on his back mounded still toward the ceiling.

Now it came to pass that Joe was no longer a patient but an employee, the transition having been so gradual as to have been imperceptible. "Joe Salvati, Iceman!" the page operator would call out, and in a few minutes, shuff . . . slap, shuff . . . slap, there would be the audible drag of that ill-favored left shoe down the corridor, and the squeakery of his wintry wagon.

Joe Salvati was king among icemen. No summons for his raw material went unanswered. Can one measure the relief that he showered in the form of ice packs, ice chips, and ice water? Because of Joe, the suppositories did not melt; because of Joe, the medications retained their refrigerated potency. Joe was Blessed Chiller to the world. For whatever reason Joe and the others worked at the hospital, it was good for the hospital, and good for them. The hospitals of that day, however, were given to low wages on the arrogant assumption that these folk were otherwise unemployable. How to pay for such devotion and earnestness? For the workers, the hospital was a haven where they could earn a living without the ridicule and rejection that was their daily measure from callous intelligences housed in more perfect bodies. Here, at the hospital, there were so many of them as to constitute a community of lovely freaks. Among their fellow oddities, they were safe and at home. To us, they were dear friends, who wore their imperfections on the outside, whilst we others kept ours well hidden and far more likely to be rotting away.

That I shall see no more that great melting mountain

behind a pushcart full of ice, the sides of the cart all hung with swinging buckets, his belt pierced with all sorts of knives, picks, and clever little saws—that I shall see Joe Salvati no more, fills me with rue. No more to feel upon my cheek, as he passed, the cool vapor that rose from his wagon in summer. It isn't fair!

Joe's wife, Theresa, worked in the hospital laundry. She was, they said, retarded. But I don't think so. Her smile was not the grin of a tickled cretin, but the still, small glee of a saint in full glory. Theresa understood linen the way few other women do. And it obeyed her the way marble did Michelangelo. Never were sheets so unstained, pillow cases so smooth, operating room towels so tidily mended. If Joe was King of the Icemen, Theresa was Queen of the Laundry. But it was Joe alone who was paged by the operator. Ice, after all, has its own importance.

For the novice intern prowling the night corridors of Saint Raphael's, to see for the first time, organizing out of the shadows, Joe and his ghastly regalia, was to have a sudden vision of Hell. Quasimodo, the hunchback of Notre Dame, must not have looked so fearsome. Within a week, however, the same sight would warm the cockles of that new intern's heart. Making his midnight rounds, the intern would hear far off an infernal clanking and that shuff . . . slap, shuff . . . slap that was the same rhythm as a heart. Perhaps that is what he was, the beating heart of the hospital set free somehow to patrol its corridors, dispensing ice as life.

"There's Joe," the intern would say to himself, and smile.

"The iceman cometh."

This hospital, no matter that it is with carpeting laid, and with reproductions hung; for all its many disguises, it is still the place where people die . . . in beds, on operating

46

tables, in cribs and incubators. From this, it has not changed in 100 years. In this building, men deliver newspapers to other men whose obituary notices will make tomorrow's news. Patient women make and remake beds, each time taking care to fold the corners of the sheets just so. On the top floor are the blind; in the basement laboratories, precisely sickened monkeys. In the ceiling above their cages, great black pipes run, carrying away gravies from slabs where water runs ceaselessly. At night, handsome black men slide giant floor polishers up and down the halls in orange parabolas of light. They sing softly to themselves as they go. And echoing through the hospital, a woman's voice intones the names of exhausted interns, summoning them to desperate bedsides. Oh, the things I have seen here which to be witness to were worth all the living that has gone before, all that is to come afterward.

A three-by-five card lies on the floor of the emergency ward. A traffic of stretcher wheels has rolled out its whiteness. Still, from where I sit at the charting desk, the card looks fresh and clean. I rise and walk to the place where the card has fallen. I pick it up. All at once, it seems as though I have turned over in my sleep and awakened.

I LOVE YOU MORE THAN I CAN SAY.

I CAN'T

The letters tremble; they wave, the two lines slanting at different angles.

My heart is pounding. For this card is suddenly a fragment that I have lifted from the surface of an ancient plain, the letters hieroglyphic, a message that waits to be solved. I carry the card into the light and brush away the encrustations of dirt, taking care not to rub out those letters. Somehow I know that what they have to tell me is . . .

Were the letters made by someone lying on a stretcher, someone who could not talk, with a head injury? Perhaps he has a tracheotomy? And perhaps, after that I CAN'T, the little card slipped out of his hand and fell to the floor? Oh, think of that, and think of despair. Or had the letters been scratched out by someone standing in the hallway, waiting for a stretcher to pass by, bearing the one for whom the letters were intended? The one who had written would have been watching for this stretcher. But perhaps it had come too soon, before the message had been finished by someone who had then to run and press it into the fingers of the one being hurried by. Or perhaps there was no stretcher at all. Perhaps, as the last word was printed, a doctor had approached. Might he have asked a question? "Are you . . . ?" Then, "I'm terribly sorry." And with that, the card slipped from the slack fingers of the writer to the floor.

I LOVE YOU MORE THAN I CAN SAY.

So! It is a passion, then. Not a father's love for a child. Nor a sister's for her brother. No, it is the love between a man and a woman that governs here. But is it a reiteration, the thousandth, of what a man already knew? Is it but the written record of speech whispered to him by a woman every night? Or is it a man's love that until now was caged, and that in this one instant, has come uncaged? Only now can it be tendered, and *must* be tendered. For it is more sustaining than all the oxygen, intravenous fluids and blood transfusions in this place. The doctors and the nurses do not know that only this little card can save their patient.

I scan the faces of the people in the emergency room. Somewhere among them is the author of that piece. I must see. I walk the length of that corridor, peering into each cubicle. I count the waiting room. I shall know at once. Such a work must correspond to the face of the one who made it.

Look! There! A woman! I knew it. She stands in the

doorway of the acute cardiac room. See how she leans forward, on tiptoe, urging something from herself into the room—an outpouring, a message. From behind the drawn curtain come the sounds of something that is hidden from her. An electrocardiograph sings, falters, sings again. There is a siffling, as of leaves. Something thumps. A silence. I shall step to her side. I shall enter that room, to see, to know. It will not be too awkward. I shall simply hold out the card to her and say, "I beg your pardon, but did you drop something?" Then I shall see flit across her face the knowledge that she has been seen, privately; that *her* heart too has been violated in this emergency room. But I make no move toward the woman. Something, a decorum, a shyness, keeps me from it. Instead, I take the elevator from the emergency room to the ward where my patients are sleeping.

It is night. I listen to the wind outside trapped in the corner wings of the hospital. It scrapes itself raw on the bricks of the walls, screaming to be let in. I listen to the wind fling itself again and again upon the hospital. Surely this place was not built by hands alone. Something other than human labored here.

There is much to be said for working at night in a hospital. One patrols intenser corridors of dedication, of love. The glare has gone out of the tending act; there is now the soft suffusion of darkness: the same hospital mirror which at noon returns a reflection far worse than the face it reflects, at night gives back only a numinous form that you can make of whatsoever you will. I suspect that, contrary to the medieval notion, night air is good for the sick body; it is certainly good for the doctor working in it, for his healing is more naturally practiced. At night, a barricade to the affections is somehow dismantled. It is at night that most people make love.

49

SARCOPHAGUS

WE ARE SIX who labor here in the night. No . . . seven!
For the man horizontal upon the table strives as well. But
we do not acknowledge his struggle. It is our own that
preoccupies us.

I am the surgeon.

David is the anesthesiologist. You will see how kind,
how soft he is. Each patient is, for him, a preparation re-
spectfully controlled. Blood pressure, pulse, heartbeat,
flow of urine, loss of blood, temperature, whatever is measurable, David measures. And he is a titrator, adding a
little gas, drug, oxygen, fluid, blood in order to maintain
the dynamic equilibrium that is the only state compatible
with life. He is in the very center of the battle, yet he is
one step removed; he has not known the patient before this
time, nor will he deal with the next of kin. But for him, the
occasion is no less momentous.

Heriberto Paz is an assistant resident in surgery. He is
deft, tiny, mercurial. I have known him for three years.
One day he will be the best surgeon in Mexico.

Evelyn, the scrub nurse, is a young Irish woman. For
seven years we have worked together. Shortly after her
immigration, she led her young husband into my office to
show me a lump on his neck. One year ago he died of
Hodgkin's disease. For the last two years of his life, he was
paralyzed from the waist down. Evelyn has one child, a
boy named Liam.

Brenda is a black woman of forty-five. She is the circulating nurse, who will conduct the affairs of this room, serving our table, adjusting the lights, counting the sponges, ministering to us from the unsterile world.

Roy is a medical student who is beginning his surgical clerkship. He has been assigned to me for the next six weeks. This is his first day, his first operation.

David is inducing anesthesia. In cases where the stomach is not empty through fasting, the tube is passed into the windpipe while the patient is awake. Such an "awake" intubation is called crashing. It is done to avoid vomiting and the aspiration of stomach contents into the lungs while the muscles that control coughing are paralyzed.

We stand around the table. To receive a tube in the windpipe while fully awake is a terrifying thing.

"Open your mouth wide," David says to the man. The man's mouth opens slowly to its fullest, as though to shriek. But instead, he yawns. We smile down at him behind our masks.

"OK. Open again. Real wide."

David sprays the throat of the man with a local anesthetic. He does this three times. Then, into the man's mouth, David inserts a metal tongue depressor which bears a light at the tip. It is called a laryngoscope. It is to light up the throat, reveal the glottic chink through which the tube must be shoved. All this while, the man holds his mouth agape, submitting to the hard pressure of the laryngoscope. But suddenly, he cannot submit. The man on the table gags, struggles to free himself, to spit out the instrument. In his frenzy his lip is pinched by the metal blade.

There is little blood.

"Suction," says David.

Secretions at the back of the throat obscure the view. David suctions them away with a plastic catheter.

"Open," commands David. More gagging. Another pass

with the scope. Another thrust with the tube. Violent coughing informs us that the tube is in the right place. It has entered the windpipe. Quickly the balloon is inflated to snug it against the wall of the trachea. A bolus of Pentothal is injected into a vein in the man's arm. It takes fifteen seconds for the drug to travel from his arm to his heart, then on to his brain. I count them. In fifteen seconds, the coughing stops, the man's body relaxes. He is asleep.

"All set?" I ask David.

"Go ahead," he nods.

A long incision. You do not know how much room you will need. This part of the operation is swift, tidy. Fat . . . muscle . . . fascia . . . the peritoneum is snapped open and a giant shining eggplant presents itself. It is the stomach, black from the blood it contains and that threatens to burst it. We must open that stomach, evacuate its contents, explore.

Silk sutures are placed in the wall of the stomach as guidelines between which the incision will be made. They are like the pitons of a mountaineer. I cut again. No sooner is the cavity of the stomach achieved, than a columnar geyser of blood stands from the small opening I have made. Quickly, I slice open the whole front of the stomach. We scoop out handfuls of clot, great black gelatinous masses that shimmy from the drapes to rest against our own bellies as though, having been evicted from one body, they must find another in which to dwell. Now and then we step back to let them slidder to the floor. They are under our feet. We slip in them. "Jesus," I say. "He is bleeding all over North America." Now my hand is inside the stomach, feeling, pressing. There! A tumor spreads across the back wall of this stomach. A great hard craterous plain, the dreaded linitis plastica (leather bottle) that is not content with seizing one area, but infiltrates between the layers until the entire organ is stiff with cancer. It is that, of course, which is bleeding. I stuff wads of gauze against the tumor. I press my fist against the mass of cloth. The blood slows. I press harder. The bleeding stops.

A quick glance at Roy. His gown and gloves, even his mask, are sprinkled with blood. Now is he dipped; and I, his baptist.

David has opened a second line into the man's veins. He is pumping blood into both tubings.

"Where do we stand?" I ask him.

"Still behind. Three units." He checks the blood pressure.

"Low, but coming up," he says.

"Shall I wait 'til you catch up?"

"No. Go ahead. I'll keep pumping."

I try to remove my fist from the stomach, but as soon as I do, there is a fresh river of blood.

"More light," I say. "I need more light."

Brenda stands on a platform behind me. She adjusts the lamps.

"More light," I say, like a man going blind.

"That's it," she says. "There is no more light."

"We'll go around from the outside," I say. Heriberto nods agreement. "Free up the greater curvature first, then the lesser, lift the stomach up and get some control from behind."

I must work with one hand. The other continues as the compressor. It is the tiredest hand of my life. One hand, then, inside the stomach, while the other creeps behind. Between them . . . a ridge of tumor. The left hand fumbles, gropes toward its mate. They swim together. I lift the stomach forward to find that *nothing* separates my hands from each other. The wall of the stomach has been eaten through by the tumor. One finger enters a large tubular structure. It is the aorta. The incision in the stomach has released the tamponade of blood and brought us to this rocky place.

"Curved aortic clamp."

A blind grab with the clamp, high up at the diaphragm. The bleeding slackens, dwindles. I release the pressure warily. A moment later there is a great bang of blood. The clamp has bitten through the cancerous aorta.

"Zero silk on a big Mayo needle."

I throw the heavy sutures, one after the other, into the pool of blood, hoping to snag with my needle some bit of tissue to close over the rent in the aorta, to hold back the blood. There is no tissue. Each time, the needle pulls through the crumble of tumor. I stop. I repack the stomach. Now there is a buttress of packing both outside and inside the stomach. The bleeding is controlled. We wait. Slowly, something is gathering here, organizing. What had been vague and shapeless before is now declaring itself. All at once, I know what it is. There is nothing to do.

For what tool shall I ask? With what device fight off this bleeding? A knife? There is nothing here to cut. Clamps? Where place the jaws of a hemostat? A scissors? Forceps? Nothing. The instrument does not exist that knows such deep red jugglery. Not all my clever picks, my rasp . . . A miner's lamp, I think, to cast a brave glow.

David has been pumping blood steadily.

"He is stable at the moment," he says. "Where do we go from here?"

"No place. He's going to die. The minute I take away my pressure, he'll bleed to death."

I try to think of possibilities, alternatives. I cannot; there are none. Minutes pass. We listen to the cardiac monitor, the gassy piston of the anesthesia machine.

"More light!" I say. "Fix the light."

The light seems dim, aquarial, a dilute beam slanting through a green sea. At such a fathom the fingers are clumsy. There is pressure. It is cold.

"Dave," I say, "stop the transfusion." I hear my voice coming as from a great distance. "Stop it," I say again.

David and I look at each other, standing among the drenched rags, the smeared equipment.

"I can't," he says.

"Then I will," I say, and with my free hand I reach across the boundary that separates the sterile field from the outside world, and I close the clamp on the intravenous tubing. It is the act of an outlaw, someone who does not know right from wrong. But I know. I know that this is right to do.

"The oxygen," I say. "Turn it off."

"You want it turned off, you do it," he says.

"Hold this," I say to Heriberto, and I give over the packing to him. I step back from the table, and go to the gas tanks.

"This one?" I have to ask him.

"Yes," David nods.

I turn it off. We stand there, waiting, listening to the beeping of the electrocardiograph. It remains even, regular, relentless. Minutes go by, and the sound continues. The man will not die. At last, the intervals on the screen grow longer, the shape of the curve changes, the rhythm grows wild, furious. The line droops, flattens. The man is dead.

It is silent in the room. Now we are no longer a team, each with his circumscribed duties to perform. It is Evelyn who speaks first.

"It is a blessing," she says. I think of her husband's endless dying.

"No," says Brenda. "Better for the family if they have a few days . . . to get used to the idea of it."

"But, look at all the pain he's been spared."

"Still, for the ones that are left, it's better to have a little time."

I listen to the two women murmuring, debating without rancor, speaking in hushed tones of the newly dead as women have done for thousands of years.

"May I have the name of the operation?" It is Brenda, picking up her duties. She is ready with pen and paper.

"Exploratory laparotomy. Attempt to suture malignant aorto-gastric fistula."

"Is he pronounced?"

"What time is it?"

"Eleven-twenty."

"Shall I put that down?"

"Yes."

"Sew him up," I say to Heriberto. "I'll talk to the family."

To Roy I say, "You come with me."

Roy's face is speckled with blood. He seems to me a child with the measles. What, in God's name, is he doing here?

From the doorway, I hear the voices of the others, resuming.

"Stitch," says Heriberto.

Roy and I go to change our bloody scrub suits. We put on long white coats. In the elevator, we do not speak. For the duration of the ride to the floor where the family is waiting, I am reasonable. I understand that in its cellular wisdom, the body of this man had sought out the murderous function of my scalpel, and stretched itself upon the table to receive the final stabbing. For this little time, I know that it is not a murder committed but a mercy bestowed. Tonight's knife is no assassin, but the kind scythe of time.

We enter the solarium. The family rises in unison. There are so many! How ruthless the eyes of the next of kin.

"I am terribly sorry . . . ," I begin. Their faces tighten, take guard. "There was nothing we could do."

I tell them of the lesion, tell of how it began somewhere at the back of the stomach; how, long ago, no one knows why, a cell lost the rhythm of the body, fell out of step, sprang, furious, into rebellion. I tell of how the cell divided and begat two of its kind, which begat four more and so on, until there was a whole race of lunatic cells, which is called cancer.

I tell of how the cancer spread until it had replaced the whole back of the stomach, invading, chewing until it had broken into the main artery of the body. Then it was, I tell them, that the great artery poured its blood into the stomach. I tell of how I could not stop the bleeding, how my clamps bit through the crumbling tissue, how my stitches would not hold, how there was nothing to be done. All of this I tell.

A woman speaks. She has not heard my words, only caught the tone of my voice.

"Do you mean he is dead?"

Should I say "passed away" instead of "died"? No. I cannot.

"Yes," I tell her, "he is dead."

Her question and my answer unleash their anguish. Roy and I stand among the welter of bodies that tangle, grapple, rock, split apart to form new couplings. Their keening is exuberant, wild. It is more than I can stand. All at once, a young man slams his fist into the wall with great force.

"Son of a bitch!" he cries.

"Stop that!" I tell him sharply. Then, more softly, "Please try to control yourself."

The other men crowd about him, patting, puffing, grunting. They are all fat, with huge underslung bellies. Like their father's. A young woman in a nun's habit hugs each of the women in turn.

"Shit!" says one of the men.

The nun hears, turns away her face. Later, I see the man apologizing to her.

The women, too, are fat. One of them has a great pile of yellowish hair that has been sprayed and rendered motionless. All at once, she begins to whine. A single note, coming louder and louder. I ask a nurse to bring tranquilizer pills. She does, and I hand them out, one to each, as though they were the wafers of communion. They urge the pills upon each other.

"Go on, Theresa, take it. Make her take one."

Roy and I are busy with cups of water. Gradually it grows quiet. One of the men speaks.

"What's the next step?"

"Do you have an undertaker in mind?"

They look at each other, shrug. Someone mentions a name. The rest nod.

"Give the undertaker a call. Let him know. He'll take care of everything."

I turn to leave.

"Just a minute," one of the men calls. "Thanks, Doc. You did what you could."

"Yes," I say.

Once again in the operating room. Blood is everywhere. There is a wild smell, as though a fox had come and gone. The others, clotted about the table, work on. They are silent, ravaged.

"How did the family take it?"

"They were good, good."

Heriberto has finished reefing up the abdomen. The

drapes are peeled back. The man on the table seems more than just dead. He seems to have gone beyond that, into a state where expression is possible—reproach and scorn. I study him. His baldness had advanced beyond the halfway mark. The remaining strands of hair had been gallantly dyed. They are, even now, neatly combed and crenellated. A stripe of black moustache rides his upper lip. Once, he had been spruce!

We all help lift the man from the table to the stretcher.

"On three," says David. "One . . . two . . . three."

And we heft him over, using the sheet as a sling. My hand brushes his shoulder. It is cool. I shudder as though he were infested with lice. He has become something that I do not want to touch.

More questions from the women.

"Is a priest coming?"

"Does the family want to view him?"

"Yes. No. Don't bother me with these things."

"Come on," I say to Roy. We go to the locker room and sit together on a bench. We light cigarettes.

"Well?" I ask him.

"When you were scooping out the clots, I thought I was going to swoon."

I pause over the word. It is too quaint, too genteel for this time. I feel, at that moment, a great affection for him.

"But you fought it."

"Yes. I forced it back down. But, almost . . ."

"Good," I say. Who knows what I mean by it? I want him to know that I count it for something.

"And you?" he asks me. The students are not shy these days.

"It was terrible, his refusal to die."

I want him to say that it was right to call it quits, that I did the best I could. But he says nothing. We take off our scrub suits and go to the shower. There are two stalls opposite each other. They are curtained. But we do not draw the curtains. We need to see each other's healthy bodies. I watch Roy turn his face directly upward into the blinding fall of water. His mouth is open to receive it. As though it were milk flowing from the breasts of God. For me, too, this water is like a well in a wilderness.

In the locker room, we dress in silence.

"Well, goodnight."

Awkwardly our words come out in unison.

"In the morning . . ."

"Yes, yes, later."

"Goodnight."

I watch him leave through the elevator door.

For the third time I go to that operating room. The others have long since finished and left. It is empty, dark. I turn on the great lamps above the table that stands in the center of the room. The pediments of the table and the floor have been scrubbed clean. There is no sign of the struggle. I close my eyes and see again the great pale body of the man, like a white bullock, bled. The line of stitches on his abdomen is a hieroglyph. Already, the events of this night are hidden from me by these strange untranslatable markings.

II

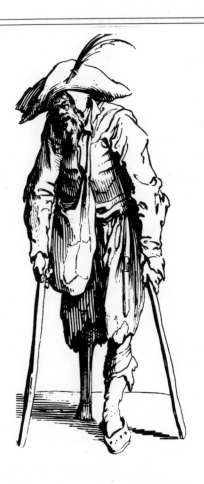

THE SPOILS OF TROY

A RIVER CASTS its influence over those who dwell upon its banks. From each river, there is given off a personal drift that is the confusion of its numberless currents, the curves and recurves of its long traipse, the strew of its bed. Even the overhanging trees, the fish within it, the swallows and gulls above, the bridges and boats, all conspire to form that special efflorescence that is the *air* of the river. It is this air that is the influence of a river upon its people.

Rivers such as the Snake and the Salmon, above which eagles hang, and from which bears prong fish, such rivers let a clarity that is reflected in the eyes of the men who live nearby. The Nile, silted up and feculent, permeates its riverlands with a listlessness that is the precursor of fatalism. And so it goes. For us who grew up by the Hudson at Troy, there was the suspicion of ill to come. Up in the hills, the hyenas were laughing. That sort of thing. Still, it was by the banks of the green-eyed, many-turtled Hudson that I learned of the resonance between a man and his river. Energy flows from one to the other and back again. In such a romance of electrons, the river-dweller becomes no other than the very tree that overhangs the bank of the stream, the weeds that tumble at its bottom, or the deep eels that lash its waters.

A man and a woman love themselves in each other; together, they become a home. A doctor gazes at his patient, and he sees himself; joined, they are one pilgrim in search of health. Just so do a man and his river become something else, a third, a confluence.

Not far from where I lived as a boy, a wooden footbridge arched halfway across the Hudson to Green Island, a dab of land midriver, inhabited only by a species of large rat. To walk across this footbridge was a very foretaste of Heaven. Had it something to do with death? So many children died in Troy in the nineteen-thirties. Tuberculosis, they said. But I suspect that monstrous irresistible footbridge.

There was so much death in the town. All those wreaths nailed to the lintels. You could not die without lilies exhaling their corruption up and down the street, the scent adhering to the skins of your neighbors like some blistering oil. And so much *handling* of corpses. To this day, it is the part of dying that I resent the most. This making free with the body, washing it, combing its hair, flipping it over to do the backside. Dragging it upstairs by its heels, perhaps, or kissing it. I do not share a tribal taste for matters funerary. Still, it ought not astonish that the survivors embrace and join not unwillingly in the rituals of death. What more tangible proof of one's own existence? He yet lives who bears the pall.

Sitting on the banks of the river, you grew used to departures, threatened and real. You watched so many pretty boats pass from view. It did not make it easier to bear.

Bobby Kinnicut was twelve when he drowned in the river. My brother Billy, Freddy Shires, Bobby, and I had sneaked off to go eel fishing. We did not see Bobby tumble. We heard only that single splash, as though a muskrat had jumped into the water. Bobby never once came up. Then we saw his empty shoe floating upside down, just beyond reach. We ran to follow it.

"I'll catch it," said Billy, "with my fishing line. Don't worry, Bobby," he called. "Here I come."

As though catching the shoe would somehow be the same as pulling Bobby out of the water; as though by some magic, once caught, the shoe would be found to contain a foot which would be attached to Bobby. And he would be saved.

"Dear God," I thought, "please let him catch it."

At the very least, the shoe was a fact that, no matter how dreadful, must be retrieved from the river, as we had retrieved so many twig boats.

Billy snagged the shoe and reeled it in. He carried it that way, swinging from a hook. Freddy and I had the eels. We ran home and rang the Kinnicuts' doorbell. Mrs. Kinnicut opened the door and sagged against it when she saw that shoe dangling from the line. It looked like a flag that had been hung upside down to announce defeat. Later, Mrs. Kinnicut told Mother that she had known the day before it happened. She had received the message in a dream, she said. Mother nodded, understanding completely. All of the women of Troy were witches then.

"How I hate that old brute," said Mother. "I wish it would dry up."

The thought made me gasp. I tried to picture the Hudson like an empty eye socket or a dry trough down into which you could *walk*, just the way you could walk anyplace. A dead gully without lilt, without sprint. What an awful thing to say, I thought. Besides, Billy and I didn't really believe that Bobby was drowned in any "all gone" or "nevermore" sense. For us he had become a kind of river nymph, wearing fish at his nose, scratching the bottom for nickels and dimes.

It was the river (I am sure of it). that made the men of Troy fight in the streets, and the women feed the pigeons. At the end of our block; where King Street and Jacob Street came together, there was a sloping square at the center of which stood a stone horse-trough. Here, two neighborhood women came to feed the pigeons. Mrs. Shires and Mrs. Russell could have been sisters, each one grayish white, plump, cooing. And each with her fringed shawl. Only their styles were different. Mrs. Shires was a shy disburser, frigid almost. From arms straight-elbowed, straight-wristed, without the least flair, she would let fall her crumbs. Having run out of grain, she would march away without a single backward glance at the frenzy she had raised. With Mrs. Russell, clearly, something else was going on. Her passionate scatterings were unbridled. Slowly at first, then faster and faster, she would cast about, hands teasing through the curtain of birds, until with a reckless pirouette, she would give up her last bit. "All gone!" she would cry, and hold up her empty hands. "See?" For a long time she would stand with the pigeons boiling about her, spattered by them, her upturned face vacant with ecstasy.

The men of Troy fought often and with the immense generosity that only the Irish bring to brawling. They held back from each other nothing of their arms, their backs, and their long bellies. Walk in Troy in the evening, and you come upon a place of special stillness. There is a ring of quiet men. Only grunts and the thud of unseen blows, the scrabbling of shoes on the cobblestones suggest the business within that ring. Nudge between the circled watchers, and you will see them. Punch. Duck. Punch. Duck. All at once, one of the two is knocked off balance.

He begins to fall, but he knows that he must not go down without pulling the other after him. Now they are rolling in bloody confabulation upon the cobblestones. These men are not ashamed to show their devotion to each other's flesh. All at once, a sigh comes from the little crowd which had hitherto been silent. It is not a sigh of sorrow or satisfaction, but rather like a mark of punctuation, a semicolon. It means that a certain point has been reached. With a single punch or kick, one of the men has gained irreversible ascendancy over the other. When you hear that sigh, you can tell who is going to win.

An hour later, you pass the tavern. You look in and see the two men toasting each other with beer. Soon, they will once again wrap around each other. This time they will sing. Outside, a woman comes with a pail and a brush. She scours the place where the cobblestones are stained with blood; then, she swings her pail to the gutter. A pink twine of scrub water races for the river.

There came the day when it was my turn. I enjoyed no great-muscled youth, but was of that frail and pallid look that is often deceptive in that it may be coincident with true good health. Barry McKenna was bigger than I by half, and with a face so handsome it seemed to have been chipped out with a clever Irish axe. He had curly lion-colored hair and green eyes. We were fourteen and in the eighth grade. The schoolyard had become a fascist pen of cement where no citizen was safe. For a long moment, we faced each other while the ring of classmates formed and clanged shut about us. There was no escape.

"I'm going to kill you," Barry said, and smiled with immense charm.

Then we closed, or rather, he bore down upon me. I raised my hands in a facsimile of boxing, holding them together lest my arms fly apart and I embrace my tragic

67

destiny. His first punch hit me on the ear, stung, then scattered. The second punch landed on my shoulder. Minutes went by. Barry punched. He danced away. I swung. It was my obligation to do so. I missed. And so it went. At last I slipped, groped for him, and we were down. I no longer had to stand and face him. He sat astride, steadying me with his thighs and belling like a white stag. Just beyond one massy shoulder, something wild and gold hovered, then broke in the air. Straining, I listened for the sigh of the crowd. When it came, I welcomed it as a bedouin in the desert welcomes the flies that are the herald of an oasis. I had only to wait a little longer.

"Aw, let him go, Barry." It was a voice from the ring.

"Come on, let the faggot go."

Above me, Barry hesitated, weighing, I suppose, the pros and cons of the suggestion. But the words of that spectator had done what none of Barry's punches could. And from the ground, I drew my fist and threw it upward. It hit him in the Adam's apple. With the other fist, I hit him in the chest over the breastbone. Barry paused, as though listening to a sound far-off, barely audible. And raising one terrible fist above my face, he brought it down . . . to his own chest, pressing. Then he coughed, and blood ran from his mouth, dripping from his chin. Again he coughed, and I was splashed with his blood. Awkwardly, like a fat cow, he disengaged himself from my body and struggled to his feet.

Again and again he coughed, each time raising new and meatier gobs of blood. I thought of Miss Cleary's cranberry conserve with which she paid Father for her bee-venom treatments. For a long moment, Barry and I stared at each other. Then, pale and sweating, he backed away from where I lay like a small creature that has been ripped and clenched, and dropped in midair. The ring of faces opened, and he was gone.

"You won," Billy said later. "You made him bleed."

"No," I said. "I didn't win."

The next week, they took Barry to the Pawling Sanatorium where my cousin Florence was a patient. First, we heard that they had collapsed his lung by injecting air into his chest.

"They're using 'pneumo' on him," said Billy. The next month they took out the upper six ribs on one side of his chest. He would have to stay in bed for a year. I tried to imagine what a chest looked like without six ribs. Something staved, dented.

"He's got a cavity," said Mother to Mrs. Fogarty.

"Ah, the poor boy. Which side?"

"Both is what I hear."

"Judas Priest! It if isn't the river, it's the chest. Is there no end to it?"

A cavity! I thought of a crater in the earth where a bomb had burst. At its base a shaggy pool where pale blind snails and cheesy beetles hopped. Creatures died in it and stank. I was certain I had done it to Barry with my fist, dislodged some essential plug that had been corking up that cavity. It was all my fault.

Near the end of the year that he was supposed to stay in bed, I saw Barry again. I had gone to visit my cousin Florence. The san was just inside the city limits, as far from the river as you could go and still be in Troy. To get to the san, you had to take the Albia bus all the way to the end of the line. From there the hospital van took the handful of visitors and the patients returning from weekend passes the rest of the way. The Pawling Sanatorium was a complex of gray-shingled buildings squatting atop the highest in a range of hills. There was a main hospital of two stories and a dozen or so "cottages" strung in a broken chain about it. There it sprawled like some loose-jointed dragon that each day demanded appeasement. Each day, one more beautiful youth. Between the river and the san lay Troy, spoiling.

The hospital van was an ancient green converted truck which was doubtless so contaminated it could have been fueled by its own germs. Billy said he could smell the fever in it.

"Don't touch anything on that bus," said Mother.

The ruts and potholes in this road just *had* to be bad for the patients, shaking loose whatever bacteria had been painstakingly herded inside rings of scar, and turning them out for yet more marauding. The driver of the van was a chronic "lunger." Now and then he would cough wetly and "raise" out the driver's window.

"He's not contagious," said Billy.

"I don't care whether he is or he isn't," said Mother. "You are not to sit near an open window on the same side of the bus."

Florence was in one of the "cottages" getting "arrested" for the second time. She greeted us with a smile.

"Guess what?" she said. "My sputum is negative."

I asked a nurse whether Barry McKenna was still there and where I could find him. He was in the main building, she said.

Barry's name was one of six on the swinging double doors. From outside the room, I could hear the ruckling of phlegm sliding to and fro in hollow bronchi. I cleared my throat and went in. It was horribly bright and sunny in that room, and every window was wide open. It had something to do with the beneficial effect of country air. Searching out Barry, I eliminated the five patients whose faces I could see. The sixth lay facing the wall, turned away from the door. A towel had been wrapped around his head like a cowl and tucked into the top of his hospital gown. I bent to peer within. What lay shrouded there was scarcely more than chin and cheekbone. But I knew him.

"Hello, Barry," I said.

His eyes, green as the river, were the only things that answered. They floated briefly up to take me in, then sank back to dead center, gazing at the wall. I made no further attempt to talk, merely stood there watching the boy who had seemed to me so big and now was smaller by half than I. As though I had wrestled with an angel all of whose mass and strength had left his body and entered mine. But the price for such a grace was that I must behold the angel as he lay dying, be marked forever by his vanishing. How dignified he looked! Like a Muslim dervish all lapped in his djellaba, who turns his face to the wall when he is ready to die.

I turned to leave. Upon the sheet, one tallow hand, the fingers each a string of polished bones. They hushed me dumb. Who could imagine that currents of warm air had ever coursed among those fingers, streamed across those translucent webs? For that hand seemed to me always to have been dead, carved from some lifeless substance and buffed smooth. All the way down that hill, I listened to the old green van cough and rattle. And I tried not to breathe.

Barry died a week later. The principal announced it at assembly. It would be nice if you all went to the wake, he said.

About the wake, three things: The coffin was open. We didn't look at each other. Barry's sister did a lot of coughing.

That evening, I walked along the river to the footbridge. I mounted the gentle ramp to the place where it went level for the long crossing. The water—very high, very black. No boat could pass under. What was that smell, sick and fenny? I had an impulse to gather twigs and start a fire to drive away whatever horrid breath was there. But I did not. Instead, I stood gripping the wooden railing, and I listened to the river gargling and spitting at the underbeams of the bridge. It was then I felt a strange urgency from my tissues to mingle with these waters, be cleaned by this river to whom one told everything, but which said nothing in return. Yes. There would be this easy leaning out into the air, a soft closing around me, above. Bobby Kinnicut was there, scoured, permeable, his hair dressed with water-weeds, charmed by the river god, and charming, sliding his moon face just beneath the surface . . .

With a haste that to someone watching from the bank would have seemed headlong, I turned and ran from that footbridge. But even now, years later, I will awaken to a tugging as of a fishing line emerging from the water. I tremble then, and I think of the river interdigitating with the town so that one could not say where the one left off and the other began, an anastomosis at the very quick of life.

IL TRAVIATO

FROM THE DAYS of my neonate, I have harkened unto grand opera. Whilst others of my ilk were lulled-a-bye to Brahms or Irving Berlin, it was to Puccini and Verdi that, crib and hammock, I surrendered. By the age of five, it had become a conditioned reflex that would remain with me all of my days. The reigning diva of Troy, New York, in the nineteen-thirties was my mother, owner of a small but truly Morphean soprano—what is now called lyric as opposed to dramatic or spinto. When she sang, it was as though a white mouse were ringing a little silver bell. Never mind that it capsized in the lower register, and whitened to a lilypontine chirp at the top, THE VOICE was ever aloft and dangerously aimed. Its effect was always the same—it put me to sleep.

Even now, instructed by some wisdom of the heart when I go to the opera, I still go to sleep. At the first bars of "Mi chiamano Mimì" or "Tacea la notte placida," a yawn rolls out of me much as thunder out of China 'cross the bay. Rarely do I make it through a recitative in a state of any but the most rudimentary consciousness. It is an affliction just this side of narcolepsy. Oft and again have I sprung to wakefulness just in time to see Tosca plunging her dagger into Baron Scarpia, or Lucia di Lammermoor still toying with the one she first inserted, then retrieved from the body of her luckless bridegroom, or Sparafucile slipping six inches of newly honed steel between the ribs of little Gilda. Is it some instinct for the meeting of cold steel and warm flesh that snaps me attentive at the first drawing of blood? Has it been these many decades of operatic surgery that urged me toward my own knifely duties?

But to sleep is, perchance, to dream. And so it is that, nodding in the mezzanine, I think to hear a voice calling out, basso profundo, somewhere in that vasty dome:

"Ché un dottore fra i presenti?"

(Is there a doctor in the house?)

It is a summons that I cannot resist. Leaping from my chair, I gallop the aisle and vault recklessly onto the stage. The house holds its breath; only a lone cello weeps on. Every eye is upon me as I nudge the sniveling Rodolpho out of the way and tend to Mimi's respiratory distress with a tank of oxygen and a mask. Quickly! A blood transfusion and two cc. of adrenalin! She must be kept going to the end of the act! On another evening, I bind up the wounds of Carmen or Cio-cio-san with a few well-placed sutures, and to each I administer a booster shot of tetanus toxoid. Ah, how these sopranos welcome my house calls, palpitating for my clever fingers, my stanchings, my unguents.

Te calma, gentle reader. I own no secret urge to stand at the operating table, strike a pose, and sing "Di quella pira" at the moment of incision. No. My only vocal performance remains a single reedy tenorial ruckus in the anatomy laboratory during the dissection of a cadaver. Just to give a flavor to the skullduggery.

It may have been the language of opera that drew me into surgery. For the language of surgery is operatic. It is Italianate, unlike the language of psychiatry, say, which is Teutonic. And just as I prefer Verdi to Wagner (we did no

German at our house), so have I ever preferred the wallows of the soma to the cooler mud of the psyche.

Take, for instance, the surgical word *choledochojejunostomy*. In fact it is something unpleasant, dire. It is the name given to an operation which hooks up the bile duct to the intestine in order to bypass an obstruction to the flow of bile. It is usually performed on people who are fatally ill, in order to relieve jaundice. It does not cure; it merely palliates. But taken as sound only, "kō-lĕh-dō-kō-jĕ-jōō-nos'-tuh-mee" is rhythmic, eloquent, sensuous. Substituted for the libretto of "Caro nome," it need suffer no embarrassment in the comparison. Esophagogastrectomy is an operation that could as well be a river. And who would not proudly wear from a chain about the neck an "arteriosclerotic heart," if sound were all. One sees it rubied, flashing from innumerable clever facets. "Incarcerated hernia," with a bit of dissection and resuturing, could be rendered as *Un Ballo in Maschera*. Imagine it: Renato appears on the stage clutching his groin and staggering about in the manner of tenors everywhere.

Renato: O mia airnia, mia airnia incarcerata!

Emilia: O ciel, ch'e questo!

Renato: Solo ora m'ange una ferita antica. (It's my old war wound).

Emilia: Quale d'averno demone ha tali trame ordite? (What demon from Hell has arranged such plots?)

In New Haven, Connecticut, where I practice surgery, many of my patients are newly emigrated Italians whose English is as rudimentary as my Italian, which is a compendium of lyric apostrophes lifted en bloc from the Italian repertory. Consider:

Angelina Esposito is seventy-eight years old. Only a week ago, she arrived from Sicily to make her home with a son and daughter-in-law. Alas, even as she was hoisted planeside from her native Palermo, her gallbladder rose up to protest this dislocation. This act of biliary treason made the maiden flight of Angelina Esposito a journey into Hell. All the way across the Atlantic Ocean, Angelina Esposito hurt. And she cursed the devil who had blackened her bile with his evil eye.

Within hours of her arrival in New Haven, the new immigrant presented herself upon my examining table, where now she lies groaning with pain. "Che avete?" I ask her. (What ails you?) From the universal pantomine of physical distress, I understand that her pain is situated in the right side of her abdomen, just beneath the rib cage.

"O madre!" I say. "Quanto soffri! Perche piangi?" (Why do you weep?)

Again and again with her hand, she indicates the place where her gallbladder lies smoldering. I, too, press the spot with my hand.

"Aie!" she groans, crescendo.

"O mio rimorso," I say.

Her silence is abrupt. She rises to one elbow, one jungly eyebrow raised suspiciously. Has something in my tremolo given her pause?

"Te calma!" I say. And I gently pull down one of her lower eyelids.

"O qual pallor!" I cry. "Mille serpi divoranmi il petto." (A thousand serpents devour my breast.)

"Eh? Che se dice?" (What are you talking about?) she grunts in the rough tongue of Sicily. I gaze upon her brown leathery face in a state of expectancy. She is Azucena, the Gypsy mother; she is Ulrica at cauldron.

As though confronted by a Sicilian scorpion, the nimble old woman leaps from my table and begins feverishly to dress, all the while keeping one black defensive eye on me and muttering what I take to be a colloquial form of male-diction, if "demon," "diavol," and "morta" are any indica-tion of the substance of her remarks.

Two days later at the hospital where I do my surgery, I see on the list of the next day's operations, the name of one Esposito, Angelina. She has been scheduled for a cholecys-tectomy, the removal of her gallbladder. And, Ah! *crude sorte!*, the operation is to be performed not by me, but by my oldest friend and most implacable rival, Mario Bracci-diferro (Arms of Steel), M.D.! *Mille serpi divoranmi il petto!*

It was the opera that did it. I should have kept to sign language. Such a wound leads me to reflect upon the word *esposito*, with the accent on the "spo." It was that rascal, that brigand Braccidiferro (Arms of Steel), who informed me that *esposito* means "out of wedlock" in the same way that *ex officio* means "having no official status." Esposito, he tells me, was the name given to each of a legion of illegitimate Italian children, many of whom eventually found their way to America. And to New Haven, Connecticut, it would seem. The New Haven telephone book lists 5½ columns of these little espositos.

The very first opera that I attended was *La Traviata*. Considering the sentiment that a man attaches to his first *anything*, and my own tuberculous heritage, it should sur-prise no one that it remains my favorite opera. To have lost one's virginity to the Lady of the Camellias, contagious possibilities aside, is a deflowering of more than ordinary bittersweetness. A perfect beginning she was, mia Violetta. More to my taste than Brünnhilde, if only in that she sports neither shield nor halberd; and safer than Salome . . . by a head. Nor is she any more a bacteriological risk than Thaïs, with whom she shares the kind of experience, riveting to the o'erswol'n imagination of a fourteen-year-old youth.

How often it is that great Art will curtain its true meaning from a less enduring audience, biding time, only much later offering a moment of revelation to the most devoted of its suitors. Like all such delayed favors, when, at last granted, the eruption of clarity is nothing short of volcanic. So it was that this year, as I sat in the opera house, watching what was perhaps the two-dozenth *Traviata* of my life, the truth was suddenly made known to me. It was as though I were seeing *La Traviata* for the first time. All at once, I knew that here was no romance of young love and beauty lost, no bacillary *Love Story. La Traviata* is really an opera about the making of a physician. For, I submit, it is Dr. Grenvil who is the central figure of the piece! Do not be misled by the brevity of his physical appearance upon the stage. All the more proof, I should think, of Verdi's genius, if any were needed.

At the beginning of the opera, Dr. Grenvil is portrayed as a rather foolish, silly man given to consorting with upper-echelon women of ill fame and their wealthy johns. In the opening party scene at the home of one of these courtesans, Violetta Valéry, the doctor is first seen exchanging chitchat with the other revelers. Violetta, of course, is a patient of Dr. Grenvil, who, it is implied, treats her for the usual disorders which are a hazard of her profession—venereal warts, pediculosis pubis, and gonorrhea. In addition, Violetta is suffering from moderately far-advanced tuberculosis. Now, Dr. Grenvil is no mere "pet" of fallen women. Neither is he a Rasputin figure, brought along to act *in loco parentis.* Nor is he meant to lend an air of respectability to the carousing. No, Dr. Grenvil is the archetypal "society doctor," himself a carouser of the first order.

So irresponsible a physician is he that when Violetta, weakened by the excitement of meeting Alfredo for the first time, suffers her famous act 1 fainting spell, Dr. Grenvil is nowhere to be seen, having already repaired to the ballroom for a little dancing after uttering such banalities as: "Yes, life is made for pleasure." "Wine is ever a friend who banishes care." "May the dawn still find us in this paradise." It is Alfredo, a mere layman, who tends to Violetta, preventing her from swallowing her tongue and, doubtless, asphyxiating. So impressed is she by his medical competence that, shortly after the party, Alfredo and Violetta agree to live together openly in a house just outside of Paris. In this, as in everything else, Verdi showed himself to be generations ahead of his time.

The next appearance of Dr. Grenvil is in act 2, scene 2, at another party. This time it is a masquerade given by a colleague of Violetta, one Flora, whose "sponsor" of the moment is the Marquis. The reasons for the party are to celebrate Violetta's return to her former life in Paris and to announce her availability to the throng of rich men present. Now, just prior to Flora's party, unbeknownst to Alfredo, his father, known as the Elder Germont, had arrived at the country retreat of the lovers and appealed to Violetta to give up Alfredo so that his sister might find a husband without the handicap of this family disgrace. The Elder Germont is a tiresome old man with a beautiful voice. In the end, Violetta cannot resist him. Sadly, she agrees to leave Alfredo and return to Paris. After her departure, Alfredo arrives, and his father informs him that Violetta has left him and has returned to her old ways.

"Mille serpi divoranmi il petto!" cries the grief-stricken Alfredo.

At Flora's party, Dr. Grenvil intercedes in a tiff between Flora and the Marquis, sings along with a band of hired Gypsies, and gossips idly about the breakup of the romance of Violetta and Alfredo. The revel is at full tilt when, all at once, Alfredo bursts in uninvited. He behaves like a swine toward Violetta, gambling recklessly, then tossing his winnings in her face as payment for her love. Violetta's response to this is another sinking spell, which, in the light of her mode of livelihood, seems a bit overstated. At the conclusion of this scene we find Dr. Grenvil joining the other guests in a general recrimination of Alfredo for his rudeness.

"Oh what a cruel blow you've struck," he sings. "Va, va, va, ne desti orror." (Go, go, go, we despise you.) Then, touched by Violetta's humiliation, Dr. Grenvil attempts to comfort her:

"All here share your grief. Dry your flowing tears. Fa cor." (Take heart).

A kindly gesture, perhaps, but hardly one that requires a license to practice medicine.

It is not until the last act of the opera that Dr. Grenvil assumes the mantle of Aesculapius, Verdi having sustained the suspense at a palpitating level. Violetta is now *in extremis* from her galloping consumption. She is living in poverty with only her maid Annina to care for her. Alarmed at the deterioration of her mistress's condition, Annina summons Dr. Grenvil despite the fact that there is no money to pay for his visit. He arrives and performs what for me is the most poignant act in all of opera. He takes Violetta's pulse. And in this single magnificent gesture is revealed the transformation of Dr. Grenvil from fop to physician. It is an understatement that Hemingway himself would have envied. We can but guess at the terrible internal struggle that accompanied it. Next, in a voice quiet, serene, barely audible, he asks,

"Come vi sentite?" (How do you feel?)

He bids her take courage. Your convalescence is not far off, he says. But Violetta will have none of his gentle deception. Doctors, she says, are liars. It is ironic that at the very moment when Dr. Grenvil undergoes his rebirth as a physician, he is publicly disputed by his patient. As if this were not enough, and here Violetta's insensitivity to the doctor's dilemma is boundless, the terminal Lady announces to the now openly heartbroken audience:

"The doctor tried to give me hope!

"Alas, with this disease, all hope is dead."

As he leaves, Dr. Grenvil levels a cold blast of truth at Annina. Violetta has only a few hours to live, he tells her, and he promises to return soon. When he does, it is to find that Alfredo and his tiresome old oom–papa have both arrived. The reunited lovers sing passionately of hope and despair. It is in this aria, "Parigi, o cara," that Violetta performs what may well be the most passive–aggressive act in all Grand Opera. She gives Alfredo a locket with her picture in it, and she tells him that one day he will marry, and that he should give his wife this picture of her as a gift. Dr. Grenvil wisely overlooks this bit of spitefulness, under the circumstances. Just then, Violetta's voice trails off and ceases. She slumps upon the bed, still cradled in Alfredo's arms. There is a terrible silence in the room. Dr. Grenvil approaches Violetta. He invites her to die peacefully. God is calling you to him, the weeping doctor sings. Now, for the second time, he lays hand upon his patient to take her pulse. But this time he feels no beat. She is dead.

"E spenta!" he says, pronouncing her so. To which Alfredo and the Elder Germont and Annina all respond,

"O mio dolor!"

In a final outburst, Dr. Grenvil demonstrates the full flowering of his compassion.

"O Cielo! Muor!" he cries. "So long as my eyes have tears, I shall weep for you."

Thus, through the death of his beautiful patient, Dr.

Grenvil regains his vocation. He is redeemed. He has become a true doctor. In light of this new insight into *La Traviata*, I propose that the name of the opera be changed to *Il Traviato*, or *The Redemption of Doctor Grenvil*.

Verdi would have wanted it that way.

WHY I LEFT THE CHURCH

Being a Sermon Delivered at the Dedication of the Hope Unitarian Church in Tulsa, Oklahoma, October 1977

WHAT A FAR CRY this from my idea of what a church ought to be. It is more than a far cry; it is a far shriek. A Jewish boyhood spent loitering in the alleys of the Roman Catholic town of Troy, New York informed me beyond the least murmur what it is that makes a church. And this, by God, isn't it. For one thing, it is too bright. All this immense wattage! As though you have somehow captured the sun itself, and given orders that it brighten the corners where you are. Light bulbs betray us, give away our arrogance and our terror. No. A real church ought to be dark, a catacomb. Did you think that prayers were eggs? That must be kept warm and well lit? No. Prayers are more like mushrooms—sweet wicked things that hatch in the dark. You let in the light, and you flush away the mystery. And where are your halos? Your wings? Your carved drapery? Where your little old women mothering the flames of candles as they fall to their knees? Why, one would think that decoration of the smallest stripe were an incitement to sin! Some of us need a bit of color, some small signpost, before we can venture along the paths of the spirit. And just look at your shameless minister without his frock on. Barbarian!

O, give me bosomy domes and spires pulled fine as taffy by the hand of God Himself.

I was twelve years old before I dared set foot in a church. St. Peter's, it was, one of the countless churches that gave to Troy, New York, during the Depression, a raised-hackle look. My Orthodox Jewish grandparents—Father's mother and Mother's father—lived with us, and had oft and again raised all the consequences of trafficking with the Gentiles. So for years, I hung at the periphery, haunted by the mysterious sparks that flashed behind those great oaken doors. I was the classic Jew, observing but not participating in the flow of history. Outside then, but close enough to catch the sensuous waftage of incense, and the nasal chanting that is the only tone of voice that works in the Christian acts of adoration and beseechment.

Incense still seems to me to be a wise choice as an offering to the gods. Unlike the carcasses of sacrificial beasts, it does not attract flies, nor does it have to be cleaned up afterwards. That incense is but the gas of prayer is attested to not only by the nose, but by the eye as well, which sees the smoke coughed piously from the swinging brazier, whilst to the ear comes the sweet muted rattle of the chain striking the little silver pot. In a moment, the air is heavy with prayer that you can hear, see, smell! Coiling, pillaring until, apse and nave, choir and spire, the whole place is saturated with the stuff. That I do not smell incense here will do you no good in the end.

For a long time, the only glimpse I got of the dark practices within St. Peter's was sidelong and occasional, taken through the great bronze-studded oaken doors, left open of an August Sunday morning. By the age of twelve, I had amassed sufficient testosterone to defy my progenitors, and, with my little Hebrew heart throbbing in my little Hebrew breast, I stepped one day across the threshold of

St. Peter's to find myself, fainting and agasp, at the very center of Heaven Incandescent. Through the arch-topped panes of stained glass, rosy, blue and violet light enkindled the worried faces of kings and shepherds, sheep and asses, each, I suppose, wrestling uncomfortably with the Trinity.

Not a foot of wall but had its saint or cross or virgin, its little herd of guttering candles. Here was St. Sebastian, looking as though he had stood up at the Alamo; there, Judas Iscariot with a guilty expression that I found strangely familiar. And that host of wax and ivory feet, at eye level, the saints having been stood up on pedestals. These were not the feet of any human being I have ever seen, but something else dead—no, *more* than dead: raised uncorrupted out of ancient graves. Some of these resurrected feet bore the dorsal wounds of the Crucifixion; others were unscarred. Each of them possessed a row of perfect even toes. A single delicate vein traversed each high and glorious instep. Of one thing I am certain: It is the pedal end of religious statuary that is the most important. Even now, on the occasion when I find myself browsing among the figurines for sale at a shrine, I can judge at once from an examination of the feet which statue is most likely to bring down blessings upon its purchaser, and which is a dud. O Sublime Podiatry!

At St. Peter's then, each saint presided over his own grotto, which was a little side-pocket in the wall, in which niche the flames of red candle-wax guttered and leapt. I do not know what the Catholics mean by the community of saints, since I have never seen a single saint that, by the least sign of recognition, admitted to the presence of any of his fellows. Like the blue bloods of Boston, they spoke only to God. Along the side walls were the stations of the cross. It was with fear and trembling that I, on that, my first day in church, joined the sad file of Irish women (where were the men?) who shuffled from one station to the other, whispering and rolling their pills. By the time I had come to Jesus Comforts the Women of Jerusalem, the seduction was complete. I was ready to convert. Yes, I would become a priest, like that one I saw way down in front, stepping backwards and forwards, with his palms apposed, doing things with a chalice and a napkin. Yes! I would be one of those. Such is the power of sacred art over the unwary.

Ah, people of Tulsa, when I think of church, I think, not of your sane unstained panes, your smooth lines, your daylight, your uncarved wood and unecclesiastic stone, I think of St. Peter's with its cool dim pillared aisles, that golden altar, that odor of sanctity, those angels fluttering high above, dumping petals, swishing garlands, blowing long golden horns, their sweet cheeks puffed in holy insufflation.

The priest mounted to the lectern. It was the time of the dreaded sermon. At some point during that morning, apparently, he had spoken with God. He had the Word. Now we were going to get it. The word that day was that this congregation of harlots and hypocrites was headed straight for Hell. I gazed about me at my fellow supplicants. There must be some mistake. These tiny gray women were surely without sin. I looked at their faces, scored with the burden of fallen husbands. Could this sparse deposit of elderly woebegone grannies and aunts be harlots? Hypocrites, maybe. But not all their exhausted souls together, it seemed, could have mustered sufficient wickedness to commit a single little venial sin, let alone the heavy mortal ones I myself was getting into. How marvelous that they could so artfully conceal their black hearts. Still, like the women of Jerusalem, the women of Troy cowered and wept, while for the next hour and a half, the priest drew such a picture of Hell as to set the jaws of a saint clacking. There were

Satan and all his tailed minions; there, the fiery plain, the pit, the snakes, the stakes, the rivers of acid and sulphur. Hell, where all was itch and sting and horrid hiss. A cold sweat rose upon the palms and brows of all of us harlots, us hypocrites. At last he was done. There was the final prayer, "Credo in unum Deum, Patrem Omnipotentem. . . ." Reckless showers of penitent coin clinked into the offering bowl. The fallen crones and I slunk toward the door. Now and then, one of them, captured by some lingering remorse, turned to cross herself and genuflect one last time.

Such was my day in church. I confess that I was, still am, seized and held fast by the sheer pomp and procession, the gaud and ceremony, the blood and wine of it. On the way out of the door of St. Peter's, I paused before the font of holy water imbedded in the wall of the vestibule. Far from being a clear and limpid pool, it looked to me sorely in need of changing. There was a quite noticeable scum upon it. But how was it to be changed? Surely no mere tap water would do. So far as I knew there was no sacred plumbing in Troy, New York, that gave forth such sparkling liquor. Surely it had to be hand-carried from Jerusalem by monks.

Attracted by the film of scum that covered the pool, I stepped closer to see, floating in the font, the little corpse of a fly, one wing raised in frantic effort at extrication. A wave of horror swept me. Here was blasphemy indeed. Here was a defilement that must be redressed. With a surge of exultation, I understood that I had been chosen (on my very first day!) to cleanse this temple, to restore it to sanctity. It was a sign! A rainbow was being aimed straight at me. I reached into the marble basin and, with trembling thumb and forefinger, picked out the fly from its turbid solution. I was about to carry it from the sanctuary of St. Peter's to the unconsecrated pavement outside. I was about to, I say, for just then Father Donahue, two hundred and fifty pounds in full cassock and surplice, bore down upon me.

"What are you doing there?" he asked in a voice such as must have been used by that bishop who ordered Joan of Arc burned at the stake.

"There was a fly in the holy water," I said. My voice was never what is termed resonant. Deep into my change of life, it was classifiably chipmunkian. "I took it out," I said, and waited for the gates of Heaven to swing open, for the grateful multitude of the blessed to welcome me in.

"Oh," said Father Donahue, with that long rising note of sarcasm, "a fly is it? Sure, and it's a fly. Anybody can see that. A fly that just looks like a *penny*." The last word boomed.

I looked again at that which I pinched. It wasn't a penny. It *was* a fly! For the first time, I realized that a person sees only what he wants to see, what he expects to see, what he needs to see. By some mysterious transubstantiation (Father Donahue was habituated to them), the fly had become a penny. And then it was that he spoke those words that catapulted me for once and for all out of the bosom of the Church.

"A boy who steals money from Jesus," he said, "will pay the trolley to Hell. Now put it back where you found it, and stay where you belong." With that, he turned on his heel and swished away. Here was a priest who could strangle a wolf with a rosary.

It was but a few steps back to the font of holy water, but it seemed a desert away. A little flick sent the insect floating once more. As I passed through the big open doors into the brilliant sunshine, I turned to see a woman standing at the font. She reached out one hand, then brought it back to dab her brow with fly water. A moment later she was down on one knee, muttering. Slowly, one at a time, I descended the steps of St. Peter's. As I left the last of them, I stuck my still-wet fingers in my pocket, and gave the first of a lifetime of skeptical shrugs.

What a sorry damp-knickers I was!

Had I then but a bit of the assertiveness with which an additional thirty-five years has enameled my hide, I should have engaged that near-sighted priest in theological argument.

It's not a penny, I should have said. It's a fly.

It's a penny, he would have insisted.

It's not.

It is.

It's not.

It is.

It's not.

Such is the caliber of most dogmatic debate. And I would have won. I never lose any of those battles. Still, with some rue my heart is laden that I never made it in the Church. Truth to tell, I still favor incantations, incense, and red candle-wax. It is certainly preferable to the hard benches of the unvarnished presbytery.

Why did I not stay in my own bailiwick, you might ask. Why did I not keep to my synagogue, my seder? Why not, indeed. Nine years of the enforced study of Hebrew had kept me from baseball after school and swimming on Saturday. I was eighteen years old before I knew the lingual pleasures of the pig, that forbidden bacon which you Unchosen fry with your eggs. Jehovah was just too easily provoked for me. Such a prickly God! Always taking umbrage, forever in high dudgeon. Just look at what he arranged for the Amalekites and how he did in Jezebel. If Lot's wife could be turned into a salt lick for a mere backward glance, why, what was coming to one who had already cast his lot with the unregenerate sinners of this world? No, I hadn't any chance with Jehovah. It was to gain relief from Divine Petulance, that I sawed my way through the bars of Old Testament Judaism for good.

But, good people of Tulsa, I have intruded upon your celebration. Surely you did not mean for me to stand here within your gallant lovely church, and natter on about my fall from grace. Forgive me. I suppose that it has festered too long in my bosom. At last the world shall know why I never go to church.

In spite of it all, I believe in miracles and in sainthood. I am not so arrogant as to scoff at these two eternal verities. Miracles I have witnessed—the dead raised, the mortally ill healed—all your standard supernatural fare. And the natural miracles too, such as what happened the time I ate a peach and threw the pit out the kitchen window. The next year, there grew a little peach tree from which a child of mine has since picked peaches to eat.

As for sainthood, well, nobody said that it was something that dwelt within a man all his life, like his bones. Rather, it is intended for most people only once or twice in their lives, and then only for a moment or two. I applaud the democracy with which God dispenses holiness, having taken the bulk of it away from those few old men and young virgins in whom it formerly reposited, and spread it about among the rest of us, so that we, each of us, Jew and Gentile, priest and prostitute, can count on being graced by at least one shaft of it before we die. One shaft of grace . . . But that's enough. For in that moment, it is given to us to know Love.

GOING NO PLACE

AT THE AGE of ten, my favorite books were the personal recountings of intrepid travelers. Most treasured was the story of a German who staggered over the Himalayas to drink yak butter tea at the Potala with His Reincarnation. Only slightly less did I love the story of that small Englishman who dined with cannibals on New Guinea, the entrée consisting exclusively of "long pig." No distant corner of the earth was left unexplored by my imagination. But I had never heard spoken aloud the names of any of these lands afar to which I made visionary journeys. And so must invent pronunciation out of whole cloth. But are we not, each of us, explorers? And do we not each plant the flag of our own country wherever we touch first foot?

I remember especially Meezo-pot-a-my´-yah. When, years later, I was cruelly ordered to corrupt this to Meh-so-pa-tay´-me-yah, you can scarcely imagine my dismay. Not a little something within me died. O Malicious Cartography that would reject Meezo-pot-a-my´-yah while printing *The Union of Soviet Socialist Republics*.

But it was to the Hē-brīdes that I longed most to go. The Hē-brīdes! It had a wild Amazonian ring. Even now, I close my eyes and see four Druid priestesses drawing magic circles around herds of men whom they keep imprisoned for God-knows-what delicious rites. Puberty is trauma enough without having to hear that one's Hē-brīdes were not such, but mere tepid Hĕh-brĭ-dēēz. Farewell to passion and dark delight.

For weeks, I hovered between melancholy and outrage. At last, the truth was revealed to me, in a dream, I think it was. They *are* the Hē-brīdes. Hĕh-brĭ-dēēz was some vulgar miscreance. I knew it then and I know it now. If you don't believe me, ask any He-bride.

Nevertheless, the linguistic shock caused such irreparable damage to my sense of geography that to this day I am unable to say for certain whether the —mania is Rōō or Rŏ.

Whoever it was that said travel is narrowing has found an echo chamber in my bosom. I like nothing better than to go nowhere. What matter the ground one treads so long as one looks up at the stars? The fact is that by the time a literate man has reached his twenty-fifth year, he is no longer able to appreciate *de novo* the charm of foreign lands. Over and over, he has visited them in books, in paintings, and in music until the minarets of Mecca are as fully realized as the paving stones of his own street. To mount a direct assault upon the far-off sights of the world would be to invite disappointment. No Orient can match the splendors of the Xanadu contrived in the mind.

I cannot comprehend the Christian tradition of mortification of the flesh. So have I, from the old couch in my study, glided over the canals of Venice, hacked my way through the vines of rural, free Brazil, and joined a caravan to Samarkand. And all without a whiff of the famous Venetian effluvium, or the propinquity of a single scorpion. My idea of horror is to be snowbound at St. Bernard's while crossing the Alps, having just spilled my tobacco pouch down a crevasse. I would sooner pass back and forth through the flames of Moloch.

Nor can I quite trust myself to do the right thing by

great monuments. Ruins unhinge me. I very much fear that, brow to stone at long last with, say, the Wailing Wall, I should find my whole attention focused upon a fly preening on my prayerbook. It was Lady Mendel, I believe, who, upon first catching sight of the Acropolis, cried: "Why it's beige! *My* color." And so might I, pinched by God-knows-what imp, utter something of equal snottitude.

In days of yore, there was more reason to go awandering and to suffer the vicissitudes thereof. One had a question to ask of the Delphic Oracle; you had to go to Ethiopia for your apes, ivory, and peacocks. Nowadays, you can buy all these out of mail-order catalogues, and Dial-an-Oracle will tell your future over the phone.

What! Restless creature, you are not dissuaded? Still would you drop arches in Afghanistan, soak through Wallabies in Bangladesh? Go then, and *vale*. My conscience is clear. *Liberavi meam animam.*

What is lacking in the tireless traipser about these planeties is a sense of place. An haberdasher dwelling *adagio* in Trenton has no business at all to intrude *agitato* upon a Mongol's hut and haggle over the price of a brass teakettle. Can the ruddy Swede, misdeposited in a Pygmy village, be anything but a source of consternation? Such a bulky wender ill fits; he is a nuisance to the little natives who must go way around him in order to do the work of their world. Whilst, *tag und nacht*, the Aryan interloper bumbles and roars and photographs. Were such an ox to contract bilharziasis from drinking the indigenous water, he would demand to be borne by the natives on a litter through the jungle to the nearest helicopter. Once back in Stockholm, he would entertain legal action against the miscreants through whose carelessness he had been parasitically infested. Oh were I a Pygmy so discommoded, I should take up my trusty blowpipe, and in the darkling forest, dip a dart and blow such a toot as would lay all of Africa mad with joy.

There is a certain easily won and false glamour about wounds sustained in the service of travel. Morris Thighs, a pudgy podiatrist from Bridgeport, pays his travel agent $2,000 in return for which he is trussed and trundled up the lower slopes of Annapurna by a convoy of Sherpas that could have kept all Asia Minor in frankincense and myrrh. No sooner is he entrusted to his own two feet, than he slips and falls victim to the impetuosity of middle age. His undoing? A grapefruit rind left on the glacier by some earlier intrepid explorer. The maladroit has now fractured his ankle. Then it is that peals of wild laughter should reverberate from peak to crag as the lofty Himalayas turn hilarious at the flopping of His Clumsiness.

Now, of course, he must be carted back down the mountain and evacuated, much as our Swede gone Pygmy-for-a-day. Just so are heroes manufactured. For months after his triumphal return to Bridgeport, he can be seen hobbling stylishly with cane or crutch toward the plantar warts of his patients, on his face the look of one who has performed impossible feats, witnessed unspeakable practices. Before such a man, other men writhe and go prone; before such a man, women gasp and go supine. So preposterously does Fortune dispense her bounties. I would remonstrate with the overly gentle Fate that decreed for him a broken leg rather than the flux of amoebic dysentery. It would tax the strongest of Bridgeportians to be asked to gaze upon the bottled souvenirs of such a retributive diarrhea. But it would be no more absurd, and, rather than adulation for his troubles, the swine would likely receive a truncheon across the shoulders.

I am fully open to the belief that the half-glimpsed yeti prowls and scurries on the slant, but I am certain that for the short time of his visit, there is no creature in all the Himalayas more abominable than Dr. Morris Thighs, Mountaineer.

As deplorable is the tourist in search of the picturesque or the sociological, who, upon his return to "civilization," hurries to his desk, drapes a wolf pelt across his lap, and writes of his experiences for the local newspaper, or a national magazine. Thus are we treated in, say, *National Geographic* to "A Sojourn Among the Visigoths" by Venerable Flesh, or "Yakking It Up in Tibet" in *Playboy*.

Travel? Like Bartleby the Scrivener, I prefer not to. I'd much rather only occasionally trek to the library or ramble through the park whose every path I know, the way a milk horse knows his morning route. Homage to Emily Dickinson who, going nowhere, went everywhere. Who can suffer gladly this dreary hauling to and fro that is the present day version of a journey? Car, train, bus or plane, one is enclosed in a compartment that is hearse-grim either out of the mistaken notion that bare utility fosters confidence in the pilot, or out of pure meanness toward the captives to the rear. Still worse are the artificial flowers, the painted-by-the-number pictures, and the piped-in music that are supposed to uplift the downcast spirit and allay anxiety, but which are none other than the phantasmagoria of nightmare. Thus pressurized, vibrating, gassed and boxed, we are swung from continent to continent much as is the bale of cotton swung from barge to pier by a grappling hook.

Despite that I go nowhere, I cherish deep within me a dream of travel by beasts and winds. What a glory it must be to join body and intent with a great animal upon whose back you sit like the top half of a centaur. As he moves, so do you, responding to the flow of flank and fetlock, feeling the thud of each hoof upon the road, and now and then bending your head over his bright maniacal eye. And what ineffable joy to hear suddenly slapped with air, the sail over your head like one wing of a hanging gull. You look up; the sail fills; it puffs; and away you skim, at once cradled by the elements and master of them. O waftage sublime . . . and unrealized. I am instantly seasick on sail or any other boat. It is the dirty work of a roughneck Fate. And I have been on horseback but once in my life, an occasion of terror for me and amusement for my former heirs, who watched and found it strangely risible that an untamed stallion should carry off at full gallop their only male progenitor. Later, the mendacious fruit of my loins were to tell it widely that the stallion was nonesuch, but an ancient sway-back whose fastest gait was a plod. Even now, though years separate me from the event, I cannot shake the memory of having been slung helpless between the dizzy mane and streaming tail of that crazed creature.

Some years ago, in the service of our country, I "trav-eled" to Korea. Of the packaging and mailing that is the army's version of travel, I shall say nothing. For to dwell upon antique discomfiture is to invite the name of whiner, and, besides, arouses no more sympathy than does the adult who publicly relives the itching of his childhood chicken pox. Once in Korea, however, with my boots deep adip in the nightsoil of the Land of the Morning Calm, I found much that was of interest and beauty—the cuckoo calling in the hills of evening, the white heron standing on one foot in the middle of a bright green rice paddy, moun-tains covered with pink jindala in the spring, thatched roofs draped with gourd vines, red oxen with their brass nose-rings. Yes, all very fine, and, I confess, seductive to the senses. But not thrilling. I found nothing there to lay trem-ulous fingertips upon my very heart, like the big yellow rock from which I dove into the sea six times a summer's day, or my own birds calling in a language with which my spirit is conversant. *My* robin, *my* dove, *my* wren. Nowhere else do they set the cobblestones just so, as at home. Nor does the light flash on any other eaves at half past five in October as my sun raises a ray in goodnight. The man who is no chauvinist about his native parts is no man to trust. He is worse than pirate, than brigand. For even such murthering devils will go limpsy-dewsy about the campfire when a song of home is raised.

What is it then that one seeks when he embarks, emplanes, boards or otherwise blasts off across the planet? To be enlightened? Ennobled? Many the returned traveler, home only long enough to deposit his acquisitions, who cannot remember where he acquired them. He holds up a tortoiseshell comb and announces quite grandly, "I bought this at a bazaar in Marrakesh." A moment later he is less certain. "Or was it the scarf I got in Marrakesh, and the comb in Tegucigalpa?" "Oh well," he says, "it doesn't matter. Just look at the work in the handle." In the mind of such a traveler, temples, statues, and hippopotami have changed location so many times that it seems *they* who have done the traveling and *he* who has remained stationary. So much has he been enlightened that he cannot be certain which ceiling it was that Michelangelo painted, that of the Acropolis or the Circus Maximus. Nor does ennoblement accrue from the venality of native merchants, or the army of petty constables who must see your "papers." Colitis tends not to ennoble. It is difficult to dwell upon *David* with diarrhea demanding otherwise. Not even Aristotle could dream high with a toothache. It is equally true that the earth is not ennobled by its trespassers. Kilimanjaro, slain by Hemingway, hardly gains elevation from the stream of its gawkers with their cans of underarm deodorant and their acreage of abandoned toilet paper.

Perhaps it is relief that the traveler seeks, relief of life, some respite from the charge of livelihood, or the lack of grace in his children. But this escape . . . is it not the same as is to be found in drink? Which is a shorter, if narrower, alley to Lethe.

There is in my neighborhood one of those delightful bars which go by the defiantly anonymous name of Tavern. It is a fitting appellation, as the place seems the very archetype of the saloon—warm, dry, and with a Rembrandt of familiar faces. It has a foggy, gaslit look. Tables, chairs, floor, and walls are all of the same dark wood. There is no art deco at the Tavern. It is the kind of bar where you can eat as well as drink. Not elegantly, but well—kielbasa with sauerkraut, franks and beans, ham and eggs, and liver and onions. All those proletarian combinations that are so apt, so dear. The food at the Tavern is footman to the beer. And the Ladies and the Gents are compassionately disposed within easy lurch of the bar as opposed to the endless holding position one must assume bladderwise whilst gadding about Westminster Abbey or the streets of Manhattan, where no man past fifty dare go without a penile clamp.

And, oh the story and song, the laughter and weeping that tunes the mind to perfect pitch. For the same reason as the traveler probes the farthest corners of the earth, so do I, moping over my vanished youth, but walk the two blocks to the Tavern where I know will be that welcome, warmth, and wine to fight off the demons Rue and Regret.

The Tavern is almost entirely without decoration, needing none. I say "almost," for, just inside the front door, between the hat rack and the umbrella stand, is one of those huge tan globes that is a map of the world. It is suspended thwartwise at the poles to a metal frame which allows for spinning. Each time I leave the Tavern, all my tissues hilarious and snug against the gloom, I give the globe a little flick to set it in motion. And all the way home I think of it spinning, out of my sight, the whole world a mere plaything within the vast dimensions of my Tavern.

IN PRAISE OF SENESCENCE

It is Tuesday, your twenty-fifth birthday. It is your lucky day. Everything good that has ever come your way has befallen you on Tuesday. So that when you awaken from sound sleep to find . . . what's this! . . . your head aching at the temples, your bones and joints stiff, your muscles sore, and a nose that pours and plashes as any freshet at monsoon, you are desolate. How can this be? you think. *It* is Tuesday. If by Tuesday, too, I am forsaken, then am I truly *abandonnato*. So run your miserable thoughts. A sense of impending doom settles over the bed in which you lie, and you arrange your aching body in a sepulchral pose.

Oft and again have I myself awakened to similar indisposition. Let me tell you what is the very best thing to do. Slide down a bit in the bed; take the edge of the sheet in the fingers of both hands and pull it up such that it conceals your face; now smile. You lucky stiff! You are a little bit sick. What, ingrate? Still you languish? Still sniffle? Wake! Enjoy! First, take two aspirin. (The headache is not as bad as you thought it was.) Present your order for breakfast in bed (anorexia is not necessarily a symptom of the disease), and settle in for a day and a night of perfect happiness. My Uncle Frank, perhaps arguing contrary to the tenets of veterinary medicine, said, "Never look a sick horse in the mouth." Never mind that the language of this aphorism be quaint; its sense is crystal clear—you've got the day off—make the most of it.

It is not altogether a bad thing to be a little bit sick. La grippe, ague, the vapors and even the common sinking spell offer to Moslem, Jew and Christian alike the chance to take to bed and to stay there while the rest of the world goes to work.

All at once you have a wave of uneasiness. What if you really are sick? What if you have made a grotesque miscalculation? You feel for your pulse. Why is it so hard to find! *How many heartbeats do I have left*, you think, and the words of Rilke creep into your mind, "Each man bears Death within himself, just as a fruit enfolds a stone." O God! You leap from your bed and run to the mirror. Should you holler for help?

But the sight of yourself in the mirror is somehow reassuring. Twenty-five! Well, well. And you stand there for a kind of quarter-century assessment. Not bad. Not bad at all. Oh there are some minor discrepancies about the face —the nose a bit retroussé, the chin perhaps unobtrusive. But, ungrateful boy, that is to carp. By any standards you are the fulfillment of a fetus's dream.

Satisfied with the externals, you stick out your tongue in the age-old fascination of man for his insides. He would peer further if he could, but it is only the tongue that is willing to be seen, flapping pink and nimble, and on the qui vive. But what is this! As you stare at it, your tongue inexplicably begins to look like something you have never seen before. It has undergone a mythic transformation. Suddenly it is jutting straight out at you, brown and coated and spiteful, like the tongue of a . . . gargoyle. You hesitate to take it back inside for fear it is poisonous. But what else can you do?

Your gaze drops from your face to the rest. Nothing amiss there. It's all the same. You breathe a bit easier. Here and there you test the fullness, the resilience, the hardness. You pinch; you cup; you weigh. But today you are no casual observer. You are intense, a terrier after a rat. That awful tongue has changed you. You search, and what you find are . . . flaws! Two white hairs, one on your chest, and the other . . . O God! Pubic! Twenty minutes more of peering turns up two small flat brown spots, each with a roughened surface. One on your neck, and the other on your tummy. You smile wanly. Is it not, you think aloud, from our very flaws, our kinks and fissures, that springs whatever becomes visible of our souls? But a gray pubic hair! O treason! All at once you hear a belch from deep inside of you. As though you contain a frog. Again, a belch: deep, reverberant and now you know that you do . . . contain a frog, that is. And instantly the whole horrid truth comes clear . . . It was the frog's tongue that you saw a moment ago! You imagine him squatting somewhere near the base of your brain, slowly puffing up his throat and coming out with that belch. You know who *he* is. He is the Frog of Death. Somehow, in your sleep perhaps, he has hopped inside of you. There is no getting rid of him. You have heard the belch of doom! Instinctively you wrap your arms about you, as if to console your flesh, reassure it that it is not so. My body, you think. My beautiful (white, black, yellow) body!

"Don't be silly," says your doctor the next day, and he laughs. A doctor who is a laugher is bad news.

"You're in your prime," he says.

You whisper a secret to him. About your hair. "It's falling out," you tell him.

"You're shedding more than your hair, my friend," he says. "A hundred thousand brain cells per day."

"Per day?"

"Per day," he says in his deep, reverberant voice. It occurs to you that he is the most repellent man you know—short, fat, bald and with dangerously bulging eyes.

"The only prime I'm in," he says, "is the prime of my senility." And he gives that terrible laugh.

Caligula, you decide, would be more simpatico than this doctor. Nevertheless, you show him your little brown spots: the one on your neck, and the other on your tummy. He bends to examine them after with a magnifying glass. He rubs his fingertip over them.

"Senile hyperkeratoses," he says. "Nothing to worry about. Little excrescences of the skin. Everybody gets them after a while."

But you have heard that word that somehow crystallizes the whole clinical picture. Yesterday you were a youth; today . . . senile!

"Fit as a fiddle," says the doctor, belching and showing his tongue.

You wish for a handful of flies to stuff in his mouth.

And bald, fat, bent, senile and mangy you flee from the doctor's office to begin the second quarter-century of your life.

Thirty-nine!

Once again to the mirror. Already the hair at your crown is scanty. A pale saucer, like some artifact long buried in the forest, emerges there. All too soon, you know, the remainder of your hair will disembed itself to commit suicide in the sink. No saucer then, but a whole platter of scalp is what you'll wear. Your flesh is no longer elastic, but flounce and wattle announce its relentless earthward decurvation. Were you Capital I? Now you are Capital S. You finish shaving and empty from your electric razor a beard dust that is pale as sand, as ash. But your beard is black! You know it is. Your hair is black, and so your beard is black. If there is order in the universe, if physics and chemistry are true . . . And then it comes to you, softly as of a tapping, tapping at your chamber door—your beard is *gray*.

And there are other losses. What was a hitherto unflagging lust has taken on a melancholy periodicity. You have loved; you have lost; you have groped for love again. You pick up a newspaper from your hometown, and you learn that a childhood friend, one of your pals, has died, leaving a grandson of his own! Your own children are large and mighty. They sweat; they swear. At thirty-nine, the days grow shorter, and night kneels like a rapist on the edge of your bed. Here and there, you die. Every hour a hundred red blood cells go to their reward, a hair follicle, another taste bud. From somewhere high above, a brain cell topples.

Forty-nine! You must hurry! Nothing about you has replenished itself. You are balder and mangier than ever, something that has been left out in the sun too long. The whites of your eyes have grown muddy; your teeth are a construct that, unsupported by metal and cement, would splinter on a sunflower seed. Peanut brittle is denied you. You brown away; you yellow off. O profligate body! Where now the streams of tears and sweat? The gallons of blood donated or shed, the white-water rapids of spermatozoa? Spendthrift Skin, how many the generations of perfect cells you have spawned and sloughed! Still, you do not miss that sweat, that blood, those tears. Of these, you have still enough. As for the spermatozoa? Well . . .

There is more. Worse. Somewhere down below, hard india-rubber lobes are mounding, mounding. It is the

Dreaded Prostate that burgeons, encroaching upon a slender little tube. Live on, and you will learn patience, my friend . . . at the urinal. You too shall stand and wait . . . and wait, and you will know bittersweet moments when urination, which was once a mere interruption of life, becomes the most exquisite of pleasures, perhaps the very reason itself for living.

That which at twenty-five was just a sapling's inkling of the oakhood to come, and at thirty-nine was a brave whistling in the dark, at forty-nine is a certainty to be faced. Of no further use a clever comb or suntan. You know . . . and you yield. That is, if you're smart, you do.

The rejuvenation of the flesh is an ancient dream. The cripple who emerged whole and pure from the pool of Bethesda is the object of wonder and envy, for he has won first prize. A loser was Ponce de León, who swilled from every river and spring in Florida and the Islands in search of the Fountain of Youth. Poor Ponce! The zealots of diet and jogging are often blind to the quality of life they would prolong. For some people, a vegetarian diet and the running of three miles a day would be a torture both exquisitely administered and endlessly endured. Physical death, in such cases, would be a technicality, one that might even be thought welcome. Robert Louis Stevenson, frustrated by the restrictions on his life caused by his tuberculosis decided that "death is no bad friend; a few aches and gasps, and we are done; like the truant child, I am beginning to grow weary and timid in this big jostling city, and could run to my nurse, even although she should have to whip me before putting me to bed."

It is not always that life is too short; it may go on too long. A visit to any nursing home, or facility for the domiciliary care of the aged, will persuade that shorter is better, what with fecal and urinary incontinence, and an absence of cognition or recognition. To say nothing of pain. Which of us would not forgo five years in such a fix for a sudden, clean and much earlier terminus? Longevity may be a Pyrrhic victory over time. I should far rather keel over at sixty, cut my losses, don't you know? Then firm and vigorous, I'd bound into the next world, ready for the Great Perhaps.

Some think to recapture youth through plastic surgery, or by lathering themselves with tinted grease, an even shallower illusion. But pissing in his shoe keeps no man warm for long. Pooh, you say, how sillily you write. And maybe I do.

The news of an artificial saliva which, if ingested, will eliminate tooth decay, renders me boggled. Whilst it would be wicked not to wish well away the ache and cavitation of candied adolescence, the prospect of a full-fanged woman of ninety-two crunching peanut brittle is too, well, ferocious for my taste. I prefer the gummy silence of Cream of Wheat. There is a certain coziness to a bowl of oatmeal that is absent entirely from a wad of taffy. Then too, the persistence of powerful teeth into great age, what with the generally recognized crabbiness that attends senescence, would surely lead to an epidemic of biting in nursing and other homes. Visiting daughters-in-law and attendants in such places would be required to wear leather gauntlets, vests of chain mail and even halberds lest they become the victims of impulsive mastication. One day there would be the inevitable reaction, and the question of defanging the aged would become like abortion, a political football.

One trouble is that you do not all decline at the same rate. Not every part of you vanishes in concert with every other part. It has proved both a delight and an embarrassment that lust remains long after the apparatus for its consummation has rusted. But if lust be the energy that drives the human race onward to new generations, then what is it doing in octogenarians anyway? Many's the brittle hip been fractured in pursuit of the phantasm that if you can fornicate at eighty-five, you are not yet old.

Not everyone acquiesces. There are those who, despite all reason and logic, simply will not go gentle into that good night. William Butler Yeats, for one, raged on. It seems that the poet, while still in his fifties, suffered a precipitous decline in his sexual potency. Which calamity, in a man who claimed that all of his poetry sprang from his rage and his lust, brought on a secondary impotence of the pen. Although Yeats continued to write, the juice and the wit had gone out of him; cool and cerebal grew the art. In the abyss of his despond, the poet moped. A friend, thinking to console Yeats with a hopeful bit of gossip, told him of one Dr. Steinach, a scientist who for ten years had devoted his experiments to the cure of sexual and spiritual impotence. His technique? The transplantation of the testicles of monkeys into the scrota of men. Yeats was more than consoled. He was intrigued. And determined at once to undergo the operation. Lovers of Irish letters everywhere tried to dissuade him from such madness. Yeats would not be put off. He would have the operation. Meanwhile, Steinach had changed his tack, and put it forth that, after all, the testicular replacement was not the essential part of the surgery. The same revivication, now claimed Steinach, could be acheived by the mere ligation of the spermatic ducts, thereby damming up the precious flow and making its creative spunk available to flesh and spirit alike.

Yeats engaged a surgeon by the name of Haire, and underwent bilateral vasectomy. No sooner had Yeats been discharged from the care of Dr. Haire than he reported to a palpitating world that he had recaptured full use of both pen and penis. The operation had been a complete success. Whilst the matter of Yeats's sexual restitution remains an article of faith, the more easily measurable of the two, his literary prowess, leaves no doubt that the operation was successful. For Yeats wrote some of his finest plays and poems in the postoperative decade. Yeats's case history has encouraged generations of aging poets. Nobody knows the burden of talent, the suffering of old poets. To what indignities, what mutilations will we not subject ourselves to warm up both art and bones grown cold?

That no such results have been forthcoming from vasectomy in this day and age is, to say the least, disappointing. I tend to think it is due to the callow indifference of urologists toward matters of poesy. Yeats was convinced that it was the Steinach operation which had saved him. Again and again he paid tribute to his benefactor. Imagine, if you will, the goaty old poet, his vasa deferentia securely tied, grinning and rubbing his buttocks on his bench. And gloating to a youthful seductee:

> *Who can know the year, my dear,*
> *When an old man's blood grows cold?*

None of this is to imply that senescence is without its joys. If you can no longer remember the names of your friends and relatives, why, you have also forgotten those of your most devoted bores, your pedants. If the ecstasy of peanut brittle has been long denied you on the grounds of precarious dentition, why, you are even further from the agony of pablum. One of the pleasures ahead of you is giving in to the temptation to mine your own past. Why would a man indulge in self-remembering, retrieving his ancient kinship with rivers and stones and narrow paths? Listen:

Forty years ago my father was a general practitioner in Troy, New York. That was before the age of specialization in medicine, and family doctors did just about everything —delivered babies, set broken legs, and removed ruptured appendixes. Despite this last, I do not think of him as a surgeon. I never watched him standing at an operating table, making an incision. But I did see him every Sunday, kneeling in his garden which he treated as though it were a ward full of patients. All day long he spent there, pruning, excavating weeds or splinting a slender stalk and marveling aloud at the exuberant swelling that bloomed at its tip. Now I am the age that he was. Then we are the same age! And now I can see what I must have seen years ago but had forgotten—his hairless white wrists submerged among the carnations, as though gripped by the lips of an incision. I do not see his fingers, hidden as they were in the foliage, busy down below, repairing the works. But I remember the air carved by bees, and the slow respiration of the trees.

Sometimes, even now, in my operating room, as I incise, clamp, ligate, and suture, I know a deeper kinship with my father. Something arcs across the decades, like a rainbow that binds the earth as if it were a gift. Why just today a red flower bloomed at the end of my scalpel: a poppy, I think. It seemed a miracle, like the leafing out of a shepherd's crook. I pinched off the bloom and tied down the stem with thread. My father was right. Surgery is gardening.

I agree with Montaigne that "to learn Philosophy is to learn to die." We start off well—with "Now I lay me down to sleep," that blend of hopefulness and sweet resignation. It ought to be recited by adults. But, not to worry. The intimations of mortality appear so gradually as to be imperceptible, like the first graying in of twilight.

Faced with the inevitable, you can do two things. You can sit in a dark room, hearkening to the thutter of snare drums, or you can adopt a good-natured posture and go about your business. The latter seems better. There is quite enough gloom in the world without your shedding more. And there is a wonderful camaraderie about aging. Come, come, little moper, look around. All the rest of us are doing it too. Except for a few liars and dissemblers. A man can lie about his age, but not about his death. It simply won't work to deny the condition to one's friends.

Think of the fun you can have drawing attention to each other's bunions and dewlaps. The trick is to find someone to get cozy with, someone to whom your warts and knobs and droopery are dear, who will understand about your bronchitic scarf. For, oh, the calmative power of love! In the profusion and prodigality of the body, who is to say where beauty lies? Some of us are drawn to footprints, which are lovely wounds in the snow.

One adores the old man who retains a touch of youth— as though the boy in him were still visible. The more one gazes on such a fellow, the younger he becomes, until the transformation is complete, and he is again that very boy of his past. Just so does one adore the young man who is early colored by age, who has felt the cool breath upon his cheek, and who has paused, listening in the night for the sound of wings.

LOVE SICK

LOVE IS AN ILLNESS, and has its own set of obsessive thoughts. Behold the poor wretch afflicted with love: one moment strewn upon a sofa, scarcely breathing save for an occasional sigh upsucked from the deep well of his despair; the next, pacing *agitato*, his cheek alternately pale and flushed. Is he pricked? What barb, what gnat stings him thus?

At noon he waves away his plate of food. Unloved, he loathes his own body, and refuses it the smallest nourishment. At half-past twelve, he receives a letter. She loves him! And soon he is snout-deep in his dish, voracious as any wolf at entrails. Greeted by a friend, a brother, he makes no discernible reply, but gazes to and fro, unable to recall who it is that salutes him. Distraught, he picks up a magazine, only to stand wondering what it is he is holding. Was he once clever at the guitar? He can no longer play at all. And so it goes.

Ah, Cupid, thou wanton boy. How cruel thy sport!

See how the man of sorrows leans against a wall, one hand shielding his eyes from vertigo, the other gripping his chest to muffle the palpitations there. Let some stray image of his beloved flit across his mind, her toe perhaps, or scarf, and all at once, his chin and brow gleam with idiotic rapture. But wait! Now some trivial slight is recalled, and once again, his face is a mask of anguish, empurpled and carved with deep lines.

Such, such are the joys of love. May Heaven protect us, one and all, from this happiness. One marvels at the single-celled paramecium, who, without the least utterance of distemper, procreates by splitting in two. One can but envy the paramecium his solitary fission.

Love is an illness and, not unlike its sister maladies, hysteria, hypochondriasis, and melancholia, has its own set of obsessive thoughts. In love, the *idée fixe* that harries the patient every waking hour is not remorse, nor the fear of cancer, nor the dread of death, but that single other *person*. Every disease has its domain, its *locus operandi*. If, in madness, it is the brain, in cirrhosis, the liver, and lumbago, the spine, in love it is that web of knobs and filaments known as the autonomic nervous system. How ironic that here, in this all but invisible network, should lie hidden the ultimate carnal mystery. Mischievous Nature, having arranged to incite copulation by assigning opposite hormones to half the human race, and sculpted the curves of the flesh to accommodate the process, now throws over the primitive rite a magic veil, a web of difficulty that is the autonomic nervous system. It is the malfunction, the deficiency of this system that produces the disease of love. Here it fulminates, driving its luckless victims to madness or suicide. How many the lovers that have taken that final tragic step, and were found swinging from the limb of some lonely tree, airing their pathetic rags? The autonomic nervous system! Why not the massive liver? The solid spleen? Or the skin, from which the poison might be drawn with knife or poultice?

Lying upon the front of each of the vertebrae, from the base of the skull to the tip of the coccyx, is a paired chain of tiny nodes, each of which is connected to the spinal cord and to each other. From these nodes, bundles of nerves extend to meet at relay stations scattered in profusion throughout the body. These ganglia are in anatomical touch with their fellows by a system of circuitry complex and various enough to confound into self-destruction a whole race of computers. Here all is chemical rush and wave-to-wave ripple. Here is fear translated for the flesh, and pride and jealousy. Here dwell zeal and ardor. And love is contracted. By microscopic nervelets, the impulses are carried to all the capillaries, hair follicles and sweat glands of the body. The smooth muscle of the intestine, the lachrymal glands, the bladder, and the genitalia are all subject to the bombardment that issues from this vibrating harp of knobs and strings. Innumerable are the orders delivered: Constrict! Dilate! Secrete! Stand erect! It is all very busy, effervescent.

In defense of the autonomic nervous system, it must be said that it is uncrippled by the intellect or the force of the will. Intuition governs here. Here is one's flesh wholly trustworthy, for it speaks with honesty all the attractions and repulsions of our lives. Consciousness here would be an intruder, justly driven away from the realm of the transcendent. One *feels*; therefore one *is*. No opinion but spontaneous feeling prevails. Is tomorrow's love expected? Yesterday's recalled? Instantly, the thought is captured by the autonomic nervous system. And alchemy turns wish and dream to ruddy reality. The billion capillaries of the face dilate and fill with blood. You blush. You are prettier. Is love spurned? Again the rippling, the dance of energy, and the bed of capillaries constricts, squeezing the blood from the surface to some more central pool. Now you blanch. The pallor of death is upon you. Icy are your own fingertips. It is the flesh responding to the death of love with its own facsimile.

Imagine that you are in the painful state of unrequited love. You are seated at a restaurant table with your beloved. You reach for the salt; at the same moment, she for the pepper goes. Your fingers accidentally touch cellar-side. There is a sudden instantaneous discharge of the autonomic nervous system, and your hand recoils. It is singed by fire. Now, the capillaries of your cheeks are commanded to dilate. They fill with blood. Its color is visible in your skin. You go from salmon pink to fiery red. "Why, you are blushing," she says, and smiles cruelly. Even as she speaks, your sweat glands have opened their gates, and you are coated with wetness. You sop. She sees, and raises one eyebrow. Now the sounds of your intestine, those gurgles and gaseous pops called borborygmi, come distinctly to your ears. You press your abdomen to still them. But, she hears! The people at the neighboring tables do, too. All at once, she turns her face to the door. She rises. Suddenly, it is time for her to go. Unhappy lover, you are in the grip of your autonomic nervous system, and by its betrayal you are thus undone.

Despite that love is an incurable disease, yet is there reason for hope. Should the victim survive the acute stages, he may then expect that love will lose much of its virulence, that it will burn itself out, like other self-limiting maladies. In fact, this is becoming more and more the natural history of love, and a good thing at that. Lucky is he in whom love dies, and lust lives on. For he who is tormented by the protracted fevers of chronic undying love awaits but a premature and exhausted death. While lust, which engages not the spirit, serves but to restore the vigor and stimulate the circulation.

Still, one dreams of bringing about a cure. For the discoverer of such, a thousand Nobels would be too paltry a reward. Thus I have engaged the initial hypothesis (call it a hunch) that there is somewhere in the body, under the kneecap perhaps, or between the fourth and fifth toes . . . somewhere . . . a single, as yet unnoticed master gland, the removal of which would render the person so operated upon immune to love. Daily, in my surgery, I hunt this *glans amoris*, turning over membranes, reaching into dim tunnels, straining all the warm extrusions of the body for some residue that will point the way.

Perhaps I shall not find it in my lifetime. But never, I vow it, shall I cease from these labors, and shall charge those who come after me to carry on the search. Until then, I would agree with my Uncle Frank, who recommends a cold shower and three laps around the block for the immediate relief of the discomforts of love.

ALEXIS ST. MARTIN

AT THAT VERY PLACE where the waters of three Great Lakes, Huron, Michigan, and Superior, come together, there humps the turtlish island called Michilimackinac. Here, in the year 1822, a shotgun was fired that blew open the body of a man and founded the science of gastroenterology. Aesculapius, the god of medicine, must have set all Olympus booming with laughter when he arranged that mayhem in Mackinac, and set in motion this unlikely Passion.

The dramatis personae are two: Alexis St. Martin, an illiterate nineteen-year-old fur trapper, one of an army of such, recruited by the American Fur Company, John Jacob Astor's corporate device with which he proposed to debeaver the forests of the Northwest and enmuskrat the women of Europe. The other was William Beaumont, age twenty-five, born of landed gentry in Lebanon, Connecticut, now an army doctor stationed at Fort Mackinac.

If St. Martin was a natural man, at home only in the trackless woods of Canada, or gliding across that country's numberless lakes on silent, home-hewn bateaux, Beaumont was the true heir of colonial solidity, a self-made man whose evenings were spent reading Shakespeare and copying into his journal Benjamin Franklin's essay, *On the Achievement of Moral Perfection.*

History is more often a chronology of accidents that befall individual men than the grand sweep of forces, or the relief of inexorable planetary pressures. So it was that on the morning of June 6, 1822, the trading post on the island of Mackinac was crowded with trappers shouting to each other in the patois of French Canada. The stench of untreated hides, piled to the roof beams, would have nauseated a wolf. Still, it did not stifle the atmosphere of exhilaration. For these "voyageurs" were waiting to be paid for their winter's harvest of fur. Later, there would be whiskey, singing, squaws, and the fighting that they loved more than any of these others. All at once, there was the stunning explosion of a shotgun inadvertently fired from a distance of three feet. One of the young men, Alexis St. Martin, dropped to the floor, blood pouring from a fist-sized hole in his left side. William Beaumont, the lone physician on the island, was summoned. He arrived minutes later and neatly extracted part of the shot from the wound, as well as pieces of clothing that had been driven inward. He then departed, with no hope for the patient's survival.

When Beaumont returned several hours later, he was astonished to find St. Martin still alive. Further debridement and dressing of the wound were carried out, and the patient was then removed to the small army hospital under Beaumont's care.

Beaumont's journal described the blast as

carrying away the integuments more than the size of a man's hand; blowing off the 6th rib, fracturing the 5th, Rupturing the lower portion of the left lung, and lacerating the Stomach by a spicula of the rib that was blown through its coat.

The surrounding flesh and clothing were burned to a crisp.
Further, he described

a portion of the lung as large as a turkey's egg protruding through the wound, lacerated and burnt, and below this another protrusion resembling a portion of the Stomach with a puncture large enough to receive my forefinger, and through which a portion of his food which he had taken for breakfast had come out and lodged among his apparel.

Each day, many times each day, Dr. Beaumont treated the wound, cutting away the devitalized bone and lung, and applying poultices "to excite local reaction." On the fifth day,

a partial sloughing took place and the febrile symptoms abated. The protruded portion of the lungs and stomach sloughed and left the puncture of the stomach plain to be seen, and large enough to admit my forefinger its whole length directly into the cavity of the stomach.

On the tenth day,

a more extensive sloughing took place. The febrile symptoms all subsided, and the whole surface of the wound put on a healthy granulating appearance . . . nature kindly performing what human foresight viewed as hopeless and professional skill might calculate upon with dubious odds. A lucky circumstance to which his miraculous survival can be attributed was the protruded portion of the stomach, instead of falling back into the cavity of the abdomen, adhered to the body wall, and by this means afforded a free passage out.

After about three weeks, Alexis was feeling quite well, and the process of scarring had begun. Despite all of the doctor's efforts, he reports that the stomach showed not the least disposition to close, gradually resembling in its appearance "a natural anus." Each time he removed the dressing, the contents of the stomach would run out.

From this point, Beaumont began to see Alexis, not on appointed rounds, but throughout the day. He observed the boy making the best of his oddness—perhaps, even, being playful with it. Wrote the doctor:

He will drink a quart of water or eat a dish of soup, and then, by removing the dressings and compress, can immediately throw it out through the wound. . . . When he lies on the opposite side I can look directly into the cavity of the stomach, and almost see the process of digestion. I can pour in water with a funnel, or put in food with a spoon, and draw them out again with a syphon. I have frequently suspended flesh, raw and wasted, and other substances into the perforation to ascertain the length of time required to digest each.

The months from September 1822 until the following May were marked by a series of abscesses, ulcerations, and sinus tracts, to each of which William Beaumont gave his daily meticulous attention. At this time, the county refused any further assistance to St. Martin, and Beaumont reported in his journal:

I took him into my own family from mere motives of charity and a disposition to save his life, or at least to make him comfortable, where he has continued improving in health and condition, and is now able to perform any kind of labor from the whittling of a stick to the chopping of logs, and is as healthy, active, and strong as he ever was in his life, or any man in Mackinac, and with the aperture still present and presumed permanent.

In 1825 there began a series of experiments performed upon the person of Alexis St. Martin by William Beaumont, experiments which were to become for the one man a magnificent obsession and for the other a hated martyrdom. Countless were the physical and chemical manipulations carried out and endured; inestimable the value of the observations made.

At what point did William Beaumont first perceive the

CONFESSIONS OF A KNIFE

possibilities inherent in St. Martin's wound? Gordon S. Hubbard, an official in the American Fur Company, was an eyewitness to the event. Years later, recalling the circumstances, he wrote:

"I knew Dr. Beaumont very well. The experiment of introducing food into the stomach through the orifice, purposely kept open and healed with that object, was conceived by the doctor soon after the first examination" in the trading post. "About this time . . . the doctor announced that he was treating his patient with a view to experimenting on his stomach."

Yet the daily entries in the medical chart kept by Beaumont give the lie to Hubbard's recollection. Would the doctor who recorded each debridement, each sloughing of necrotic tissue, each happy mound of new granulation tissue, would he be likely to harbor the secret hope that the wound would *not* heal? That all of his surgical efforts would fail?

Where lies the truth? Perhaps there are no "facts." Perhaps all of history is conjecture, interpretation, and, in the end, faith. Doubtless Beaumont's recognition of the importance of the wound to science was early. Why then, all the more honor to him who left no stone unturned in his meticulous efforts to bring about the healing of it. Since history fails to inform absolutely in this critical matter, one is left to one's own interpretative devices. I prefer to think of Beaumont as tortured by his conflicting desires: to keep the wound from healing, and to ensure that it healed. I like to think that Beaumont struggled with his temptations and overcame them. That in the end he behaved as a good doctor would: His patient's well-being came first. The fact that the wound did fail to heal may be thought of by incurable romantics as a kind of divine retribution for having behaved irreproachably.

And so the experiments were begun.

Imagine, then, Alexis. He reclines on a cot, naked to the waist, ordered to lie on his right side for hours at a time while the inserted material is digesting. Then ordered to lie on his left side that the gastric juice might run the more freely, be the more easily collected. Then asked to carry the vials of this fluid in his armpits so as to achieve for it the body's temperature. All these things he is commanded to do day and night and many times each day. Now see William. Approaching the bed whereon the other lies, he pauses at his table to select a hollow reed for insertion. He peels the stopper of lint from the orifice of the wound, and hastens to catch the fluid in his vials. His face is a study in earnestness. Having made his measurements, he sits at his desk, recording the data, amounts, temperatures, stages of digestion, in his notebooks. All this while, Alexis must lie still, or he must fast, or eat only certain foods. And all to a purpose whose significance Alexis cannot comprehend, and that for him has no importance at all.

How much does a man owe to another man who has saved his life? Does he owe him the remainder of his own?

Nowhere in the countless retellings of this story is one invited into the heart of Alexis St. Martin, young, well muscled, and strong as he has often been described, homesick for his lakes and forests, despondent, not permitted even the automatic pacing that is the prerogative of the caged leopard, but coerced into lying down, even as that leopard, *couchant, regardant*. His keeper, the man who *saved his life*, ties a string around the piece of meat that Alexis *knows* is coming, knows that the other man is going to poke into his body. With what a sign of resignation does he raise his left arm out of the way, the better to proffer his wound, the better to submit again to the intrusion that is for him a kind of rape. How can he know that Beaumont is never more alive than when he is pursuing him. That, even as he, St. Martin, mopes, Beaumont is exhilarated, expectant, buoyed by the hope of discovery?

Implicit in the word *voyageur* is the intention to return home. Without this expectation, the voyageur becomes an exile. For Alexis, the house of Beaumont is a place of exile, a wild island upon which he has been cast by a roughneck fate. And just as he is an innocent prisoner, so is Beaumont a jailer both benevolent and sightlessly cruel. William Beaumont has given back to Alexis St. Martin not his life, but the mere appearance of it.

But eventually the spirit of Alexis St. Martin began to suffocate. Having been strung and pipetted and measured beyond endurance, he bolted back to the woods and lakes of his homeland. Wrote Beaumont in a letter to the publisher of his experiments:

I regret very much that it is not in my power to offer more varied and satisfactory results, but, unfortunately for me . . . he has absconded and gone to Canada, at the very time I was commencing a number of more interesting and important experiments upon the process of digestion and power of the gastric liquors, and I very much fear I shall not be able to recover possession of him again. He was unwilling to be experimented upon, though it caused him but little pain or distress.

For William Beaumont, the defection of St. Martin was no less than the thievery of his dreams, the petulant act of a stupid ungrateful boy. He would get him back if it was the last thing he did.

The year was 1825. Such was St. Martin's vaunted frailty that he had easily managed the solo journey back to his native Quebec, a distance of two thousand miles, in an open canoe. For the next two years, William Beaumont wanted only one thing: he wanted the "ungrateful boy" back. In desperation he appealed to the officers of the American Fur Company, asking them to be on the lookout for him, and, whatever the cost, to bring him back. At last, word! From one of these officers who reported that the ungrateful boy was now married to an Indian woman, and living in the country, "poor and miserable beyond description." Two years later, at the urging of a petty constable, Alexis returned to Beaumont accompanied by his Indian wife. During those four previous years, Alexis had worked hard to support his family, as a voyageur for the Hudson Bay Fur Company. All this time he had remained robust and well.

From 1829 to 1831, St. Martin and his wife lived at the home of Beaumont and his wife in a sort of "Upstairs, Downstairs" arrangement. The second set of experiments were carried out. And Alexis acted as servant to the Beaumonts, chopping wood, carrying bundles. During this time, he also fathered more children, working toward his grand total of seventeen.

That these second experiments, too, were impeccable, flawless, and simple, is a matter of fact.

Experiment No. 34
March 14, 1830
At 8 o'clock 15 mins. introduced two ounces of rare roasted beef, suspended by a string, into the stomach, and at the same time put one drachm of the same kind of meat into twelve drachms of gastric juice, contained in a vial, and put it into his [Alexis's] bosom. The piece in his stomach, examined every hour til 12 o'clock, . . . exhibited a uniform but very slow process of digestion, confined entirely to the surface of the meat. In four hours about half of it only was dissolved and gone. That in the bosom, at the same time, digested still slower, owing probably to the circumstances that the fluid in the vial had been taken out when the stomach was in a morbid condition, and had been

permitted to get cold, even to the freezing point. This last circumstance, however, was probably of less importance than the other. The meat in the stomach was too much confined by the string, was not permitted to move about freely in the gastric fluids by the natural motions of the stomach, and consequently did not digest so fast as it otherwise would have done. Another circumstance or two may also have contributed to interrupt the progress of digestion, such as anger and impatience, which were manifested by the subject during this experiment.

One can hardly be surprised.

Alexis left again in 1831 and returned in 1832, at which time Beaumont, skittish over the possibility of permanent separation, attempted to bind Alexis to him with a legal contract.

". . . And the said Alexis covenants and agrees to submit to, assist and promote by all means in his power such Physiological or Medical experiments as the said William shall direct . . . on the Stomach of him, the said Alexis, either through or by means of the aperture or opening thereto in the side of him, the said Alexis . . . and will obey, suffer and comply with all reasonable and proper orders . . ."

in return for which Beaumont agreed to pay St. Martin the fee of $150 "for the service of a year."

For a period of ten years, Alexis intermittently endured and fled. For ten years Beaumont experimented or pursued him. Here, then, are the appearances of what happened. Whether they constitute, in fact, the realities is what makes the study of history no mere memorialization of events or the handing down of sacred prejudice, but a subject open to interpretation by thoughtful men and women.

Why tell once more this oft-recounted story of Beaumont and St. Martin? It is the best known, most beloved tale in all of American medicine. Beaumont's experiments, crude but meticulous, have long since entered the living literature. Beaumont himself is most securely elevated and enshrined. Everywhere there are Beaumont rooms, tablets, portraits, memorabilia. Everything but a constellation in the heavens, and over this only Aesculapius has jurisdiction. It is precisely to recast this event in terms truer to the dear and faulty nature of man that I here conjecture anew.

There are risks in such an undertaking. A profession that fails to pay homage to its heroes will surely fall on hard times. Not so long ago heresy was punishable by burning at the stake. Still, let us dare.

And so, two men, one the son of Congregationalist landed gentry in Lebanon, Connecticut: solemn, moral and dutiful down to his Yankee bones; the other a carefree child of the Canadian backwoods: strong, wise in the way of the forests, his mind uncluttered with literacy or other unnatural contrivances. Whilst Beaumont read Shakespeare, Pope, and Robert Burns to while away his time, and even copied Ben Franklin's essay *On the Achievement of Moral Perfection*, Alexis learned to traverse the woods as silently as an Indian, to trap muskrat and beaver, to fight with his fists, and to drink whiskey. Who is to say that wisdom lies at the end of one path over the other? It were an arrogance to ascribe to either one the role of the model man. They were . . . what they were. That it was Alexis who lay blasted open on the floor of the trading center, the recipient of the skill and professional devotion of William, and not William lost and helpless in the depths of the trackless forests of the Northwest until Alexis should happen by to lead him to safety, that such was the turn of events is the accident of fate.

Two men. Neither one noticeably graced with a sense of humor. The one grimly following his purpose, self-righteous, pious; the other a roisterer grown morose through a lifetime of invalidism and pain. A feisty cockerel doomed to the tireless chaffing of his fellows who called him "the man with the lid on his stomach." What, for God's sake, did they talk about all those hours and days and weeks and years while they lived in service to The Wound? While Alexis reclined on a bed, and William sat next to him, dangling his infernal string, or inserting his little tube? Did they tell each other jokes? Make up stories? Play word games? Did Alexis undertake to teach William the patois of French Canada? Did William teach Alexis chemistry? Was there any affection between them? Any love? Or were they two self-serving con artists, each out for his own; Beaumont for fame and glory, St. Martin for the money to buy liquor? Was it just Beaumont buying and Alexis selling? A sullen ten-year commerce in gastric juice?

The idea for the experiments once having seized Beaumont, it was never to turn him loose. It was as though the doctor himself had been seized between the jaws of that wound, and that it was, in fact, Alexis St. Martin who kept William Beaumont in thrall. Alexis had long since become the grail after which Beaumont was to yearn for the rest of his life. For Beaumont the Measurer, there was a magical exhilaration in the adventure. Once having stepped through the mangled portieres of St. Martin's body, he was never to look back. Not Orpheus on his way to Hell owned such a feverish expectancy. What was his anguish when again and again he was halted, turned back by the capricious petulance, the coquetry, the recalcitrance of St. Martin?

For every man there is one single enterprise that describes his life, and that makes of all that went before, all that is to follow, mere anticipation or recollection. For some it is the selection of a mate, for others the death of a child, for still others the consummation of a passion, be it for God, woman, fame or power. For Beaumont it was the experimentation that he conducted upon the person of Alexis St. Martin. Never mind that the event was that which happened to St. Martin, and that Beaumont's role was but to seize upon it and to turn it to his purpose. What kind of man was William Beaumont?

Such a man was able to write to the absconded Alexis, encouraging him to leave his wife and family "for only two years." It could not possibly be a hardship, he wrote. And, yet, though Beaumont had himself experienced the love of a wife, the joys of fatherhood, he did not shrink to ask another man to forgo these companies. At last, he offered him more money. Beaumont demanded of St. Martin that he earn his livelihood by selling his body for the glory of science. As well ask an agnostic to take a little bag of whips out into the desert to mortify his flesh for the glory of God. Is Beaumont aware of the true nature of his role as pimp and libertine? When offered the choice between martyr and whore, it does not astonish that St. Martin opted for the latter, more easily comprehending himself as a commodity than as a sacrifice.

How much does one man owe to another man who has saved his life? Does he owe him indentured servitude for the rest of his life? His undying and daily manifested gratitude?

By 1832, Beaumont was famous, the darling of the medical world, and the pet of the surgeon general. Alexis, now twenty-eight, "dark hair, dark eyes, dark complexion and five feet, five inches tall," was drinking heavily. In many of the ensuing 116 experiments done between 1832 and 1833, Beaumont reported evidence of this: "The diseased appearance of the stomach was probably the effect of intoxication the day before."

On and on they battled, Beaumont to "procure," "secure," and "gain control of" his laboratory animal; St. Martin for his freedom from the demonic doctor who, he must never forget, had *saved his life*. "I am determined to [complete the experiments] if I even have to shut myself up with Alexis in a convent." Again and again, they part only to come together. It is as much a reflection of Alexis's loyalty as it is of Beaumont's personal magnetism.

But here, in 1834, is Beaumont writing to the surgeon general after still another jilting by the elusive St. Martin.

"I know well his disposition and his ugliness, and hope rightly to defeat them." Beaumont resolved to forgo any attempts to retrieve St. Martin, but to wait until such time as

he will have spent all the money I advanced him to provide for his family for the year ensuing, become miserably poor and wretched, and be willing to recant his villainous obstinacy and ugliness, and then I shall be able to regain possession of him again, I have no doubt.

Add a horrible leer, and some hand rubbing, and presto, Fagin the Viper.

By 1846, Beaumont, having been separated from St. Martin for a decade, is undeterred in his efforts to get him back. He learns that Alexis has given up drinking, that he is in good health, and that several of his children have died. Letters were exchanged, those of Alexis being dictations to which he affixed his sign.

This from Alexis, "You who are a married man and a father, can easily conceive how very difficult it is for me to tear myself forcibly away from here without a reason for doing so."

And this from William:

You know the embarrassment and interruption that have occurred heretofore to the prosecution of my experiments upon you

on account of having your family with you. . . . I can conceive
no difficulty, unreasonableness, or cruelty in leaving your family
comfortably situated and provided for with their friends for the
short space of a year or two, while you came to fulfill your
obligations to me faithfully and honestly.

And again from Alexis: "I am happy where I am. I can
earn sufficient to support them here. Money is of no object
to me alone. My only wish is to see my family satisfied."
Now, who can blame Alexis St. Martin for adding to this
statement of sweet reasonableness: "Several medical men of
Montreal have asked me to hire to them for that purpose,
but I did not decide . . ."

As late as 1852, Beaumont the Wily is appealing to the
better nature of his guinea pig.

Mon ami:

. . . Alexis, you know what I have done for you many years
since; what I have been trying and am still anxious and wishing
to do with and for you; what efforts, anxieties, anticipations and
disappointments I have suffered from your nonfulfillment of my
expectations. Don't disappoint me more, nor forfeit the bounties
and blessings reserved for you.

Beaumont was furious. Elsewhere he comments:

This's just for a snatch of Monsieur's ways, thus goes he on in
tricks and *lies,* and thinking to get well paid for it.

He never saw Alexis again.

William Beaumont died in April 1853. He had fallen and
struck his head the month before. The cause of death was
sepsis emanating from a carbuncle of the neck. Even with
Beaumont safely in Heaven, Alexis St. Martin was pursued
by his doctor's ghost in the form of Sir William Osler, who

endeavored to obtain permission for an autopsy to be performed, the famous stomach to be retrieved for the Army Medical Museum in Washington. In this he was foiled by the peasant cunning that had oft and again proved the exasperation of Dr. Beaumont. Outraged by the suggestion of the autopsy and determined to prevent its occurrence, the family of the little voyageur "kept the body at home much longer than usual and during a hot spell of weather, so as to allow decomposition to set in and baffle the doctors." By the time of the funeral, the body was in such an advanced stage of decomposition that it could not be admitted to the church, but had to be left outside.

Two men. As bloodless as a stick, Beaumont subjugates his passions. He will do good for mankind, and wend not his way to the fleshpots. It is one of the sublime ironies that, with all of his good intentions, it was precisely toward the rarest fleshpot in the world that William Beaumont turned. Once having arrived, the dazzled doctor's hunger could not be assuaged by a lifetime of probing and stringing and instilling. St. Martin becomes the noble savage, the bearer of the Miraculous Wound, which sets him apart from all other men. But St. Martin does not remain the virginal creation of Beaumont's Puritan dream. Alexis's own concupiscence is at last aroused. Soon he becomes what he must, the virgin turned whore, selling himself bit by bit, drop by drop to his assiduous purchaser, asking higher and higher prices for his services, turning petulant and surly when denied, a wily peasant now rather than a fresh-eyed savage. He would coax from the landed gentry every last bit of payment that was his due. Thus did St. Martin, daily stoked with wads of bacon by the scrupulous, minute, self-taxing Beaumont, fall from innocence.

Was William Beaumont really bloodless in his unending violation of Alexis St. Martin's civil rights? Or did something else, besides his obsession for discovery, goad him to assume the role of hunter, with Alexis St. Martin as his pelted prey? Consider the language of metaphor which Beaumont employs in his descriptions of the wound. Again and again, he compares it to a mouth, or an anus, and finally to a "half-blown rose." To a lover, the beloved and all his parts are beautiful. For one three-year period, Beaumont forsook his family to travel with St. Martin, to Washington, to New York, to consultations with such authorities as Benjamin Silliman. A longed-for journey to Europe with Alexis failed to materialize. During this time another 116 experiments were conducted. From 1832 to 1835, Beaumont lived away from his family, and with Alexis.

If one is to invoke Aesculapius as the prime mover of these events, and Artemis, goddess of the hunt, as his henchwoman, in that it was she who contrived the endless flight and pursuit of the two, is it not possible that Aphrodite, she of the seafoam, was equally conspirator, inflicting unrelieved passion upon the luckless Beaumont. Was William Beaumont gay?

What! Hear Beaumont pleading with Alexis to stay— just a little longer—stay, for I need you? See the distraught doctor clinging to the defiant St. Martin who wrenches free, leaving a torn shirt in the heartbroken Beaumont's grasp, as his beautiful wound-bearer plunges from the hated house into the woods for which he hungers, the lakes for which he thirsts? No. That would be to make of this story a romance, a legend, to give it a grand significance that it does not deserve.

That Beaumont was a passionate man is illustrated by an incident involving a matter of honor, the original insult of which has been lost. A certain Lieutenant Richards announced that Beaumont was no gentleman. Beaumont retorted that Richards was a liar, a base villain, and a poltroon. If vituperation alone be the measure, why Beaumont is clearly the victor. Beaumont further showed his mettle, if not his common sense, by challenging Richards to a duel in order to settle the affair. Richards refused to receive the letter of challenge, reiterating haughtily that he would not accept unto his hand the communication of a man who was so patently not a gentleman. Whereupon Beaumont circulated a public announcement that Richards was indeed those three things which he said he was in the beginning . . . a liar, a base villain, and a poltroon. Oh well. But it does leave the reader of biography with a piquant mystery —why was Beaumont, in the eyes of Richards, no gentleman? Was their altercation over a woman? Unlikely, given Beaumont's singleness of purpose. Was it over money? Unlikelier still. Was it a difference of opinion over Beaumont's treatment of a case? Perhaps. The age-old boredom of military life has been known to reduce even the most elegant men to indignant capons, the one demanding satisfaction and the other not deigning to condescend. Or, shame on me, had Beaumont touched the dark underside of life and Richards been witness to it?

A man of passion, then, himself, how is it that Beaumont was blind to the passion of Alexis St. Martin? They could not have been friends. Friends, by definition, consider the emotional needs of one another. Remember the tone, sulky and severe, in which Beaumont insisted that Alexis leave his family for two years.

It is no wonder that, in the end, St. Martin, no longer naive, squeezes cash from his user, penny upon penny, and then one penny more. By just such dunning does he announce his very existence. It is necessary to him. He *must* believe that he is getting back a little of his own.

As if to show in the end that he knew something that Beaumont did not, St. Martin survived his doctor by twenty-eight years. What cheek!

PAGES FROM A WOUND
DRESSER'S DIARY

I AM A DRESSER of wounds.

My name is William. My beard is grayer than it is black, but I am childless.

I make my rounds on the decks of the steamboat *January*.

I dress the farmers who make up the regiments of Tennessee, Ohio, and Kentucky. I plant my acreage of gauze, then stand back to wait for the dark red fruit to appear.

The *January* runs from Pittsburgh Landing to St. Louis, taking on casualties and carrying them north to the great hospitals. Sometimes we stop for stragglers who have made it to the banks of the river, lone soldiers who wave their arms and call out to us. Their urgency is spectral. To them we are no fat asthmatic auntie, but a musicked barque drawn by dolphins.

We are a hospital boat. We are also a pest house and morgue. We freight typhoid and tuberculosis and measles as well. At night we stop to bury the dead along the banks. There are two coffin makers aboard. They are very busy. At night, I lie in my berth and feel the river slapping against me. It is more Styx than Mississippi. I am more Charon than William.

The things I have seen on this river.

I have seen two drowned men hustling each other along

the current, jostling, glancing off, rearing up over rocks and shoals, as exuberant as boys racing downhill.

I have seen rats swimming among planks of ice.

I have seen a horse and rider lying half submerged at the bank so that only the head of the man and the hind parts of the horse are visible, a centaur that had lost its way, its beautiful nostrils gone knobbly with rot.

I have seen the sleeping bellies of soldiers, soft as the bread women bake.

I have seen that path of moonlight on water for which there is no word.

Say that a man is missing a finger. So forever after he is known as "Fingers." It is a peasant wisdom that invents a man from what he does not have. There is a fine accuracy to such nicknames; I call this river "Bridges," for it has hardly any. Chug away an entire day, two even, and you do not see a bridge.

But when there is one, there is that long anticipation from the instant it is sighted far ahead, the exultation when at last the sun is carved from view and . . . hush! You are *in*, a quick narrow place that is cool and green and dark. How reluctantly you emerge from such an arcade into heat and light, all the usual affairs of August.

This Mississippi unspanned is no place to be.

Two Rebel boys among the day's haul. Their eyes are covered with blood-stained cloths tied around their heads. Side by side, they sit on a bench, waiting. I untie the bandages. I saturate the dressings with water, and only when they are heavy with the water do I dare tease away the cloth from the underlying tissues lest I pull away valuable flesh. Once. Twice. Three times and four I lay bare . . . no eye, but an empty socket at the base of which puddles a yellowish ichor. One burst globe droops from its stalk upon the cheek below. A snip of the scissors, and it, too, is gone. The boy is startled by the sound.

"What was that?" he asks.

"Nothing," I say, "a bit of dead flesh. Something you didn't need anymore."

But vision is too cunning a thing to be killed by the putting out of eyes. It were an arrogance of anatomists to believe it so. No, vision is a nomad. He'll tent where he can —in the knees, the hands, the groove at the back of the neck. He will peer from behind the bars of rib cages, watching, and seeing no less than were he in his proper sockets.

Dawn. In the pilothouse. We have been at river for an hour. A dozen crows have stayed the night in a great cottonwood tree that looks like clackety Death with his graspers out and waving. The crows hunch one to a branch, sawing at the air and working each other into a rage. As though beckoned, the community lifts. One after another dislocates his wings and flaps off, twelve black rags shaking away to God knows what ghastly food. For crows, this is the land of plenty. A blind peck at the earth will yield some morsel of new flesh.

It has begun to rain. A passionless fall that is unlikely to spend itself imprudently and so will persevere all day. A dead man is sighted on the bank. The crows have seen him too. Already the vanguard is grounded and stepping close. I rush with two others in the small boat to do the burial. One man rows, and we others shout and wave our shovels at the crows. We race them for the prize. The birds pull at their work until we are within arm's reach. Only then do they hop sideways a bit, sizzling to get back. The soldier's face is gouged, one wrist ripped, tendons unstrung.

But rain has filled his open mouth and runs across his chin. Who would imagine that from this fixed scream such a limpid brook could run? His papers state that he is Secesh from Mississippi. We dig in the mud and lay him in. It is far too wet for a grave. In three days he will seep into the river and the fish will have him.

I don't know why we think that's better than crows.

Our cargo is typhoid, and worse by far than the most terrible battle wounds. These men bed in their excrement, too weak to raise themselves from where they lie. Most are doomed by the time they are carried aboard. There are so many, I cannot tend them all. I pour a few drops of midnight whiskey upon their black tongues and listen to their breathing. Some are pricked by a sudden delirium to spend their last caches of strength in wild careering about the deck. One man rises abruptly from his pallet and, as though chased, runs to the railing, calling out in tongues. Before he can be restrained, he has thrown himself over the side.

A man lies down to die. He sweeps a man-sized space of the deck, wraps himself in a blanket, turns half a circle and, doglike, settles to the boards. The wounded lie about among the dead, indistinguishable from them save for the occasional hand reaching upward to retrieve a beloved something that floats just away and away. So shyly, so gently do men die, that I found myself having just injected one man, a calico printer from Georgia, only to discover that he was long since cold and lifeless. An hour before, I had heard him swapping accounts of the battle with his fellows.

Even the *January* is ailing. It is hard to write, the old nanny quakes so.

A bend in the river is a risk. What will be around it? New horror? Or more of the same horror? At three o'clock, standing at the railing of the upper deck, I see a lone woman on the west bank. I could not be more overcome by the sight were she some species of ape. She stares at the steamboat. As we draw abreast of her, she raises one hand and waves. It is the most tentative, the wariest of gestures. In the same manner, I wave in return. We are neither of us soldiers. Merely, we hope not to be shot.

This morning I amputated the leg of an Illinois farmer, a man of forty-five years. We have run out of chloroform, and it must all be done without. I had hardened my heart for screams, but the man made no single sound. Now and again, I looked up to see was he conscious. He was. Once he opened his mouth as if to cry out, but . . . he merely yawned. There are such men who bear a legging bravely, as though bravery were the best in human character. But I think this kind of courage redemptive only in a wicked man, for in him it stands forth like a beacon in a wild gray sea. I would sooner trust a man who owns more honest tissues, who would not hesitate to shriek and bawl. Even Jesus wept. Not to unleash the throat in such circumstance is to misunderstand the natural purpose of outcry which is twofold: to comfort the uncomfortable with the sound of your own voice. What could be better proof that you are still alive? And to summon aid from all within earshot.

Still, as the leg of the Illinois farmer fell free and was lifted away by the orderly, the fellow raised his head to gaze after it. Once, in the woods, I came upon a snake in the midst of his shedding. And a neat, deliberate job it was the serpent did. Yet even as he slithered off, the creature turned to gaze one last time at the sad transparent crumple on the ground.

Midnight. I sit at a small table on the covered deck. All about me in close neat rows lies the sick freight. A thick fog obscures all but my pen and notebook. The light of my lamp is turned back upon itself by the mist it cannot penetrate. The darkness is absolute. To the left of me a man coughs, then spits. Nearby, a rattling breath, caught on a bolus of phlegm, hesitates. For a long minute it ceases. I hold my own breath. At last I hear it again, and we breathe. Here and there the involuntary flux of dysentery sputters. Forlorn cracklings, the untranslatable fragments of a lost language. I may one day forget the words and deeds of this time, but I shall never rinse from memory the sound of a man turning into watery stool, his own mass diminishing as the puddle of his excrement widens and spreads until . . . the transubstantiation is complete.

"Oh, Jesus," someone cries.

And flowing beneath these sounds the low ceaseless murmuring of three hundred men drifting in and out of private dreams. I cannot tell where their whispering leaves off and the whispering of the river begins.

Strange shapes gather in the exhalations of dying soldiers! These are jets of vaporized pain shot from the wounds themselves. No mouth could make such air. Above the cots, currents hang, opaque with memories of battle. Now and then, budged by some impalpable breeze, they commingle, then part, then roll together in a thunder soundless and profound. I gaze, and kindle into dreams. I see Shiloh. I hear the hornetry of working muskets in the peach orchard, shouts, and the brave bugle blowing hullabaloo.

All at once, there is a scream—a blend of bell and cannon. It rings with majesty. I look across the field to the peach orchard, and see . . . Pegasus galloping through the trees. He is riderless, and his famous wings are beating at the dazzled air. Again he neighs! The spaces are not large enough for him, and his wing tips bruise against the stubborn branches. No orchard could contain him. Now he rears and sets his feathered parts in motion. They are impossibly high, arched, grabbing air to their undersurfaces, gathering it into gusts, churning it into a wind to rise upon. But he does not go aloft. He cannot. Again he rears, and now I see the bayoneted belly, that dark slit through which presents, like half-delivered twins, a double loop of pinkest bowel.

Fifty, no, a hundred yards he races, sidestepping, straining, his great boxy teeth biting at the peach blossoms, then stops, and, as though at his prayers, kneels into the horse pond at the edge of the orchard. The wings of Pegasus are broken. They flap with the sound of dry straw. It is a creaking. At last they come up, like the sleeves of a kimono drawn across the velvety nostrils. Bubbling, the great horse lies on his side, showing the whole fall of his intestines. He is everywhere soiled with blood.

Overhead and all around, the flowering peaches.

Headache. All day the boilers hammering and the crepitation of muskets. We shall be deep imbrued by nightfall. The men say there is no ground uncovered by a fallen body. One strides them like a carpet, they say. Yesterday I counted twenty-seven bullet wounds in a single corpse.

I feel myself being taken over by the river. Soon I shall be more catfish on the prowl than man. I tell this to Mr. Forbes, the pilot. He laughs. Mr. Forbes is a huge man with a red beard that makes him appear both calm and wild. I judge him to weigh no less than 250 pounds. He knows every crook and turn in the river, just when it will turn peevish and throw up a snag, or a sawyer.

"If I thought," he says, "this war was to put a stop to slavery, I should not lift a finger to check the rebellion. The children of Ham are to be slaves for all time."

Just then a deck hand calls out a sounding.

"How is the river today?" I ask him.

"Low," Mr. Forbes says, and smiles. "Don't worry," he continues. "When it runs dry I can tap a keg of beer and run four miles on the suds."

Old lady *January* is sick and undergoing surgery at the Cairo dock. Rupture of the boiler, I am told. But the way she coughed all the way to Cairo, I think pneumonia has set in too. Now she lies nuzzling the levee, sniffling rope, and waiting for the doctor.

At the St. Charles Hotel, we are in hearing distance of the guns. The hotel has been commandeered for bivouac, and everywhere there are soldiers recounting and bragging and deploring the generals. Now and then, a man will display his souvenirs, a sword or regimental flag. The streets are sodden and throng with men walking, just walking, all aimless in their motion. A cavalry officer gallops by, sending up gobbets of mud from the hooves. Everywhere there are wagons, munitions. In the main square, I see a stand of a thousand rifles.

I drink a whiskey at the saloon of the St. Charles, and go down to the levee to watch the repairs. I cannot keep my distance from that boat and that river. The short while I am ashore, I am on alien land. The customs are exotic, the language unintelligible. In the berth next to the *January*, the *Paris C. Brown* is being loaded with bales of cotton. Fifteen blacks, barefoot and stripped to the waist, work the cargo from one another in a line.

> *Ole roustabout ain' got no home.*
> *Makes his livin' by his shoulder bone!*
> *Oh I whoop my woman and I black her eye*
> *But I won't cut her th'oat kaze I skeered she might die.*

Up sack! You gone.
Up sack! You gone.
N'Yawlins niggers ain' got no sense.
Up sack! You gone.

Coonjine songs. They would tempt back all my dead.

A fourteen-year-old fifer has been taken aboard. His brow has been torn away by a minié ball, and his right thigh is fractured. He has pale yellow hair and blue eyes. I carry him from the litter to a cot, and his head falls against my chest. Suddenly I feel myself to be a comet hurtling through the sky.

The boy shudders. I follow his gaze to my hands where the fingernails are edged with old dried blood. Who can blame a boy for shuddering at the claws of an old bear?

Now and then, one of the other men will start to sing. Soon he is joined by another, then another, until a great tuneless chorus rises.

I listen, and this whole world of men becomes for me a pantry that is rattled by the river until, one by one, the cup handles slip their hooks, and each china plate falls its little fall, and shatters.

If it were not for the chloroform, I could not do it, amputate the arms and legs. I have not the stomach nor the heart for this hacking. Last night I probed the neck of a boy to retrieve a minié ball that had got lodged next to his great artery, the lantern held by a man barely able to stand. Each time I got near to dislodging the pill, the boy screamed out, "Jesus, help me," and each time I felt like Pontius Pilate.

Two of the new amputees have got the rigors. It is horrible to watch them struggle to unlock their jaws for speaking. Their eyes are thrown upward in staring, their necks and spines so arched and rigid that only the back of the head and the remaining heel are in contact with the bed. Finally, awake to the very end, they strangle in convulsions.

Here, Death, you beauty, you outdo yourself.

Another dawn. I stand on the upper deck. A strange elation has seized me, so that I am unable to sleep, except fitfully. The *January* rocks at her pier to the rhythm of far-off Minnesota springs. It is a soothing, amniotic pulse. On the opposite shore, a great hairy cypress surmounts the stream, dangling tendrils in the water.

Scouts have warned of the approach of two Rebel rams, and we waddle up the Yazoo River for a distance of ten miles to hide. The rams are steamboats that have been fitted out with steel beaks at the prow. They are for goring.

The Yazoo is nimble and narrow. We huff against her current in our haste to get hidden. A few miles upstream, we see a great solemn rising in the middle of the river. It is the tilted hulk of a half-sunken steamboat, an old corpse, I know, from the shroudage of creepers that drape the upper deck and wind into the pilothouse. These river-lands of the South are everywhere red with such ulcerous ruins, all their chugging done, then banged out in a great flame as the boilers burst and exploded. Still, this corpse has kept something of itself, some boathood, calling to mind better days, with tapered banners notched at one end, and harmonicas playing in the saloon, and bales of cotton piled on the deck. A silence falls as we pass. On a tiny island that is no more than a yard of sand, a great blue heron stands, one leg folded upon its breast. Boatmen and water birds have the same dreams.

Still we lie sequestered among the vines of the Yazoo. Elisha, the fifer boy, lies upon the deck as though carved into the wood. I spend much of my time sitting by him, listening to his childish tales of the battle. How bravely he must have marched beside the drummer, tootling his fife. Were I a Tennessee soldier, I would have followed that sound into death. And so his elder brother did.

At noon today, he begs me to carry him to the edge of the deck so that he can look down into the water. I do, and lay him face down at the railing, lifting and holding him so that he peers straight down along the side of the vessel. He is delighted to see his reflection in the still water.

"Take off my bandage," he says. "I want to see my wound."

"No," I say. "Why would you see your wound?"

"Because I want to see what I have suffered for my country."

I unwrap the gauze from his forehead and hold him once again over the side of the boat. Looking down into the Yazoo, we can see the avulsion of his brow. It cannot be stitched, so much tissue having been torn away. Elisha studies it. And as I gaze with him down into the river, I see in the water behind his head the yellow noonday sun. There is the great red star-shape on his forehead, and, behind it, the sun. For a moment, I cannot say for certain. Is it the wound that hangs in the sky and the sun that blazes between the eyes of the boy?

The men have caught an alligator and keep it below the deck in a box that the coffin makers have made for it. It is the river god, they say, and as long as we've got him on board, the *January* is safe from the Rebel rammers. Sometimes in the evening, when they feed it a rat, I hear the jaws snap shut. The sound carries to the deck where the sick men lie, and it makes them smile to think of the fun of it.

How bored the men are. When they hear the sounds of battle, they grow eager and hot eyed. Like a horse kept too long in its stall will chew the wood of the barn for want of something to do. Those that are able crawl out upon the uncovered deck to feel the sun. Elisha lies among them. The men offer him bits of candy, little presents, a whittled stick. They ask him to play his fife for them. But he has not breath enough. What shall I do?

The Union ram, *Queen of the West*, has been ordered to the mouth of the Yazoo to clear the way for us. We saunter off behind her. An hour later, what excitement! The Rebel stegosaurus, *General Leighton*, is waiting. The *Queen of the West*'s beak took the *Leighton* squarely on the guards twenty feet back of her stern, cut through her like a ripsaw, clove her timbers apart, pierced her entrails. The dark waters rushed madly into the hull, and she settled rapidly. But the wounded *Leighton* gripped the beak of the *Queen* and held fast to pull her conqueror down with her. The *Queen* backed off, and the two vessels ground and wallowed past each other like churning giants, the sinking *Leighton* taking on water like a thirsty sailor. Full speed! Within minutes, we can no longer see the men of the *Leighton* floundering in the river. We won!

Once again, we are heading downstream toward Pittsburgh Landing to pick up a load of wounded. Elisha's fever rages. The wound has begun to stink. One of the coffin makers has been carving for him a pair of crutches out of a Rebel flagstaff. I am impatient for them, asking the man again and again, "Aren't they finished?"

There are three hundred sick and wounded on the middle deck. Overnight we have become a barge smeared with shit from typhoid and dysentery. From below, there is the ceaseless hammering of the coffin makers. Each day, dozens of these men die, and each night we bury them along the banks, the graves hurried scoopings in the earth. On the next trip we will be reminded of our haste when we see poking from the earth some portion of an uncoffined body, an arm groping, a leg dancing up into the sunshine. If waking from the dead is as painful as this dying, I'll have none of the Resurrection, thank-you.

It is three years that I have ferried the dead over these dark waters. A terrible sameness discolors my days. It is as though the river has turned upon itself, taken its tail into its mouth to make a circle around which I am doomed to chunter. How I long for something . . . a waterfall! Yes, a cataract. Oh let me imagine it! At first a drubbing, barely audible; then a quickening of the stream. The noise rises, a thunder greater than the hum of these miles of cliffs along the bank. I look ahead and see that the river has ended, all at once, in blank open space. The *January* captured and pulled along. We tilt; we hang; we plummet. Ah, there is an end to it! In a cloud of wrack and lovely foam!

The boy will let only me dress his wound. Sweet tyranny! He cannot read nor write. I write down a letter to his mother.

Dear, kind Maw,

I have been brave, but I have sinned greatly. I hope that the sinning will not win over the brave part when the time comes soon to be chosen for Heaven. I thank you for your prayers. I am sure they will help me.

Your boy Lishe.

He has been with me for four weeks. I have kept him with me. He begged me to keep him with me. I have forgotten how it was he came on board. But it must have been like Moses out of the bulrushes. Sometimes I take the notion that the slattern *January* and I are man and wife. And it is upon this old squaw that the boy Elisha was begot. When he is able, he plays "Yankee Doodle" on his fife for the men on the deck, and they lose their last bit of fluid in tears.

One of the wounded is a Rebel lieutenant from Alabama. There is a sucking wound in the left side of his chest. With each inspiration, air is expelled through this ragged opening despite that I have plugged it with oiled lint. His fever rages. He is dying, certain. I sit with him during his final hour, and, all the while, he talks of the reasons for the war, why it is necessary.

At the last, he tears a brass button from his gray coat and places it in my hand. There is that telltale "give," the taut arms gone limpsy, the onrush of silence that fills the space abandoned by labored breathing, moans; and I, visiting such new silences every hour.

Prisoners released from a Rebel jail. So thin that the origin and insertion of each muscle is visible. The bony eminences all but burst through the skin. Only one man is hugely fat. He is but slightly wounded—a bullet in the buttock. I shall have to dig for it, I suppose. His corpulence is an insult to the others and to me that must go after the pellet. I watch the fat man manage the boarding plank. He grunts and puffs like a cow in a barn. They say some are eating human flesh.

What is this that gathers in me as I watch the boy struggling to die like a man and cannot? A kind of madness that urges me to kill him, to save him from death. A caged animal will kill its young. Is it to save it from the long death of captivity that the bear takes up her cub in her jaws, shakes it, and dashes it against the bars?

It is a day of amputating, dressing, and pronouncing death. In the midst of it, I am told by an orderly that Elisha has died. Near the end, the boy called out for me. William! William! although he never called me anything but Doctor. It was the delirium, the orderly said, but I was not there to see that. For me, now, these many "Williams" are the urgent whispers of love. How quickly in war love springs full grown—at least as fast as death. And how gently the one falls into the other. He is to be buried with the others this night. The gravediggers promise to mark the spot.

In the evening I watch from the deck as the coffins are unloaded and carted up the bank. One of the crutches I have given to be placed upright alongside the grave. The other I throw into the river. Now I accompany the coffin up the bank. I stand over it as the grave is dug. I gaze down at the coffin, then bend to stroke it, to feel, not boy, but board.

Later, from the deck of the *January*, the hillock is starred with the large fireflies that cloud in these parts, making it appear to me, far below, that the entire bank lies already in the sky. I stand at the railing until that burglar, night, has finished stealing from me the gravesite of that boy. I turn back toward the deck where the wounded lie. The odor of a rose would suffocate me, the color of sky madden. I hate every lovely thing. Let me hear screams and weeping. I begin to dress a wound, a soupy crater in the flank of a man too old by far to have fought in any war. "A vulture would turn me down," he says. He shakes with fever; I could light a match to his skin.

I probe the putrid depths of the great sore. The man

shudders to feel me there. My finger meets the hard blunt tip of a minié ball. I fish it out and hold it up for the man to see. Very faintly, he smiles. All at once a strange feeling comes over me. It is happiness. I cannot resist it. And I know that if love came once, it may come again. If love should not come, still I know why I am alive.

THE MASKED MARVEL'S LAST TOEHOLD

MORNING ROUNDS.

On the fifth floor of the hospital, in the west wing, I know that a man is sitting up in his bed, waiting for me. Elihu Koontz is seventy-five, and he is diabetic. It is two weeks since I amputated his left leg just below the knee. I walk down the corridor, but I do not go straight into his room. Instead, I pause in the doorway. He is not yet aware of my presence, but gazes down at the place in the bed where his leg used to be, and where now there is the collapsed leg of his pajamas. He is totally absorbed, like an athlete appraising the details of his body. What is he thinking, I wonder. Is he dreaming the outline of his toes. Does he see there his foot's incandescent ghost? Could he be angry? Feel that I have taken from him something for which he yearns now with all his heart? Has he forgotten so soon the pain? It was a pain so great as to set him apart from all other men, in a red-hot place where he had no kith or kin. What of those black gorilla toes and the soupy mess that was his heel? I watch him from the doorway. It is a kind of spying, I know.

Save for a white fringe open at the front, Elihu Koontz is bald. The hair has grown too long and is wilted. He wears it as one would wear a day-old laurel wreath. He is naked to the waist, so that I can see his breasts. They are the breasts of Buddha, inverted triangles from which the nipples swing, dark as garnets.

I have seen enough. I step into the room, and he sees that I am there.

"How did the night go, Elihu?"

He looks at me for a long moment. "Shut the door," he says.

I do, and move to the side of the bed. He takes my left hand in both of his, gazes at it, turns it over, then back, fondling, at last holding it up to his cheek. I do not withdraw from this loving. After a while he relinquishes my hand, and looks up at me.

"How is the pain?" I ask.

He does not answer, but continues to look at me in silence. I know at once that he has made a decision.

"Ever hear of The Masked Marvel?" He says this in a low voice, almost a whisper.

"What?"

"The Masked Marvel," he says. "You never heard of him?"

"No."

He clucks his tongue. He is exasperated.

All at once there is a recollection. It is dim, distant, but coming near.

"Do you mean the wrestler?"

Eagerly, he nods, and the breasts bob. How gnomish he looks, oval as the huge helpless egg of some outlandish lizard. He has very long arms, which, now and then, he unfurls to reach for things—a carafe of water, a get-well card. He gazes up at me, urging. He *wants* me to remember.

"Well . . . yes," I say. I am straining backward in time. "I saw him wrestle in Toronto long ago."

"Ha!" He smiles. "You saw *me*. And his index finger, held rigid and upright, bounces in the air.

The man has said something shocking, unacceptable. It must be challenged.

"You?" I am trying to smile.

Again that jab of the finger. "You saw *me*."

"No," I say. But even then, something about Elihu Koontz, those prolonged arms, the shape of his head, the sudden agility with which he leans from his bed to get a large brown envelope from his nightstand, something is forcing me toward a memory. He rummages through his papers, old newspaper clippings, photographs, and I remember . . .

It is almost forty years ago. I am ten years old. I have been sent to Toronto to spend the summer with relatives. Uncle Max has bought two tickets to the wrestling match. He is taking me that night.

"He isn't allowed," says Aunt Sarah to me. Uncle Max has angina.

"He gets too excited," she says.

"I wish you wouldn't go, Max," she says.

"You mind your own business," he says.

And we go. Out into the warm Canadian evening. I am not only abroad, I am abroad in the *evening!* I have never been taken out in the evening. I am terribly excited. The trolleys, the lights, the horns. It is a bazaar. At the Maple Leaf Gardens, we sit high and near the center. The vast arena is dark except for the brilliance of the ring at the bottom.

It begins.

The wrestlers circle. They grapple. They are all haunch and paunch. I am shocked by their ugliness, but I do not show it. Uncle Max is exhilarated. He leans forward, his eyes unblinking, on his face a look of enormous happiness. One after the other, a pair of wrestlers enter the ring. The two men join, twist, jerk, tug, bend, yank, and throw. Then they leave and are replaced by another pair. At last it is the main event. "The Angel vs. The Masked Marvel."

On the cover of the program notes, there is a picture of The Angel hanging from the limb of a tree, a noose of thick rope around his neck. The Angel hangs just so for an hour every day, it is explained, to strengthen his neck. The Masked Marvel's trademark is a black stocking cap with holes for the eyes and mouth. He is never seen without it, states the program. No one knows who The Masked Marvel really is!

"Good," says Uncle Max. "Now you'll see something." He is fidgeting, waiting for them to appear. They come down separate aisles, climb into the ring from opposite sides. I have never seen anything like them. It is The Angel's neck that first captures the eye. The shaved nape rises in twin columns to puff into the white hood of a sloped and bosselated skull that is too small. As though, strangled by the sinews of that neck, the skull had long since withered and shrunk. The thing about The Angel is the absence of any mystery in his body. It is simply *there*. A monosyllabic announcement. A grunt. One looks and knows everything at once, the fat thighs, the gigantic buttocks, the great spine from which hang knotted ropes and pale aprons of beef. And that prehistoric head. He is all of a single hideous piece, The Angel is. No detachables.

The Masked Marvel seems dwarfish. His fingers dangle kneeward. His short legs are slightly bowed as if under the weight of the cask they are forced to heft about. He has breasts that swing when he moves! I have never seen such breasts on a man before.

There is a sudden ungraceful movement, and they close

upon one another. The Angel stoops and hugs The Marvel about the waist, locking his hands behind The Marvel's back. Now he straightens and lifts The Marvel as though he were uprooting a tree. Thus he holds him, then stoops again, thrusts one hand through The Marvel's crotch, and with the other grabs him by the neck. He rears and . . . The Marvel is aloft! For a long moment, The Angel stands as though deciding where to make the toss. Then throws. Was that board or bone that splintered there? Again and again, The Angel hurls himself upon the body of The Masked Marvel.

Now The Angel rises over the fallen Marvel, picks up one foot in both of his hands, and twists the toes downward. It is far beyond the tensile strength of mere ligament, mere cartilage. The Masked Marvel does not hide his agony, but pounds and slaps the floor with his hand, now and then reaching up toward The Angel in an attitude of supplication. I have never seen such suffering. And all the while his black mask rolls from side to side, the mouth pulled to a tight slit through which issues an endless hiss that I can hear from where I sit. All at once, I hear a shouting close by.

"Break it off! Tear off a leg and throw it up here!"

It is Uncle Max. Even in the darkness I can see that he is gray. A band of sweat stands upon his upper lip. He is on his feet now, panting, one fist pressed at his chest, the other raised warlike toward the ring. For the first time I begin to think that something terrible might happen here. Aunt Sarah was right.

"Sit down, Uncle Max," I say. "Take a pill, please."

He reaches for the pillbox, gropes, and swallows without taking his gaze from the wrestlers. I wait for him to sit down.

"That's not fair," I say, "twisting his toes like that."

"It's the toehold," he explains.

"But it's not *fair*," I say again. The whole of the evil is laid open for me to perceive. I am trembling.

And now The Angel does something unspeakable. Holding the foot of The Marvel at full twist with one hand, he bends and grasps the mask where it clings to the back of The Marvel's head. And he pulls. He is going to strip it off! Lay bare an ultimate carnal mystery! Suddenly it is beyond mere physical violence. Now I am on my feet, shouting into the Maple Leaf Gardens.

"Watch out," I scream. "Stop him. Please, somebody, stop him."

Next to me, Uncle Max is chuckling.

Yet The Masked Marvel hears me, I know it. And rallies from his bed of pain. Thrusting with his free heel, he strikes The Angel at the back of the knee. The Angel falls. The Masked Marvel is on top of him, pinning his shoulders to the mat. One! Two! Three! And it is over. Uncle Max is strangely still. I am gasping for breath. All this I remember as I stand at the bedside of Elihu Koontz.

Once again, I am in the operating room. It is two years since I amputated the left leg of Elihu Koontz. Now it is his right leg which is gangrenous. I have already scrubbed. I stand to one side wearing my gown and gloves. And . . . *I am masked*. Upon the table lies Elihu Koontz, pinned in a fierce white light. Spinal anesthesia has been administered. One of his arms is taped to a board placed at a right angle to his body. Into this arm, a needle has been placed. Fluid drips here from a bottle overhead. With his other hand, Elihu Koontz beats feebly at the side of the operating table. His head rolls from side to side. His mouth is pulled into weeping. It seems to me that I have never seen such misery.

An orderly stands at the foot of the table, holding Elihu

Koontz's leg aloft by the toes so that the intern can scrub the limb with antiseptic solutions. The intern paints the foot, ankle, leg, and thigh, both front and back, three times. From a corner of the room where I wait, I look down as from an amphitheater. Then I think of Uncle Max yelling, "Tear off a leg. Throw it up here." And I think that forty years later I am making the catch.

"It's not fair," I say aloud. But no one hears me. I step forward to break The Masked Marvel's last toehold.

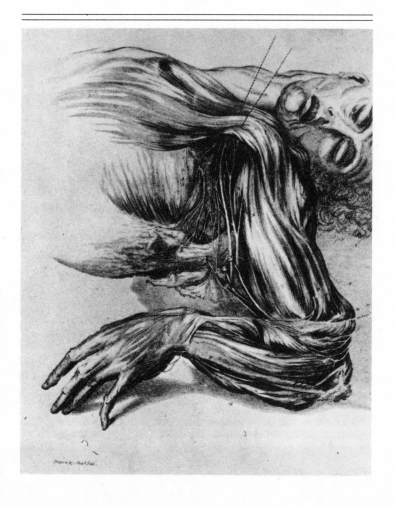

TUBE FEEDING

A MAN ENTERS a bedroom. He is carrying a lacquered tray upon which stands a glass pitcher of eggnog. There is also a napkin in a napkin ring, a white enamel funnel, and an emesis basin. In the bed a woman lies.

It is eight o'clock in the morning. Precisely as he turns the knob of the door, she hears the church bells. At the sound, a coziness comes over her. There is nothing more certain than that he will appear, when he is most needed, when everything is ready. She has been awake for two hours, considering the treason of her body. But now that is over. She feels privileged to have known ahead of time of his coming, as though it were an event that had been foretold to her. She smiles up at him.

"Lovely," he says, and smiles. He carries the tray to the nightstand near the bed and sets it down. He bends then to kiss her head which is almost bald from the chemotherapy.

"What's lovely?" she asks him.

His smile broadens.

"The morning. Breakfast. You."

"Just lovely," he says again as she knows he will.

He opens the drawer of the nightstand and, after a moment of hesitation, selects a silk scarf. He holds it up.

"This one?" he asks.

She nods. He folds the scarf into a triangle, places it across her forehead and ties two ends of it at the back of her head. He tucks the folds in at the sides with a small flourish. He has become adept at this. Even now, after so many weeks, he marvels at the smallness of her head. It is so tiny and finely veined, no more than a pale knob, really, or a lamp of milk glass etched by the suture lines of the skull.

Before the chemotherapy, she had had dark brown hair which she sometimes braided into pigtails. It had given her a girlish look that amused him until he read somewhere that people who were dying of a lingering illness often took on a childlike appearance. Thereafter he wondered whether a long dying was really a slow retracing of life until the instants of death and conception were the same.

Hours before, she had opened her eyes to see him stepping into the room to give her the dose of pain medication. The moonlight streamed where he stood, an arc of blackness carving the moon of his face in half, hiding the lower part from her view. She wondered what he was thinking then. She thought it might possibly be like what she felt as a child when she picked the crumbs out of her grandfather's beard as he slept.

That was several hours ago. There would still be time before the pain returned. He could always tell when the pain was beginning to come back. Almost before she could. Her eyes took on a glitter that was a presentiment of the pain. All along he had considered the pain to be a mistake on the part of her body. Something had gone awry, been derailed, and so she had the pain. It was the kind of mistake that was an honest piece of ignorance by a person he loved. Between the long prairies of pain, there were narrow strips of relief when the dream of health was still given to her. In these intervals she would lie as on hillocks of cool grass, having caught at last, among her fingertips, the butterfly for which she had such nostalgia.

The man sits, one buttock on the bed, his legs arranged for balance.

"Ready?" he asks.

She nods. He never seems to notice the great red beard of tumor that, having begun in her salivary gland, had grown until it fills, now, the space between her face and her chest. There, where once her neck had been, she is swollen to bursting. Like a mating grouse, she thinks, or one of those blowfish. It is as though there is a route which his mind obeys, carefully, so that he sees only her brow where the skin is still pale and smooth, nothing below her eyes. She was someone who had always counted appearance for so much. Her own looks had stood her in such good stead. After all, she would say to him, I caught *you*, didn't I? And then came the cancer which, if it had only remained internal, hidden, would have kept for her the outline of her self. But this tumor had burst forth, exuberant, studding her face, mounding upon her neck, twisting and pulling her features until she was nothing but a grimace trapped in a prow of flesh.

"I look like Popeye," she said once.

He had not smiled.

The man rises, then kneels playfully beside the bed. To the woman, he seems taller in this position than he had while standing. As though, in the act of folding, he had grown. Kneeling *is* the proper posture for prayer, she thinks.

Now the man stands again. He folds down the sheet to the level of the woman's hips. Her abdomen is scaphoid, like an old boat which had been pulled up onto the land long ago, its mast and appointments pirated. Still, in the bend of each rib, there was retained the hint of wind and bright water. From the left upper quadrant of her abdomen, from what looks like a stab wound, there hangs a thick tube of brown rubber. The end of the tube, some eighteen inches from the skin, is closed off by a metal clamp, a pinchcock. The number *34* is stamped in black on the tube, announcing its caliber. The man takes the stiff tube in his left hand, letting it ride across his fingers. He removes the white gauze pad that has been folded over the open end and secured there by a rubber band. Always at this point, she feels that the act is exploratory, as though they are children left alone in a house, and have discovered for the first time how to do something mysterious and adult, each needing the assurance of the other.

The man releases the pinchcock. A few drops of mucoid fluid drip into the emesis basin. Sometimes there is a little blood. He is relieved when there is none. He wipes the end of the tube with the napkin and inserts the nozzle of the calibrated funnel into the gastrostomy tube, setting it firmly lest it slip out during the feeding. They look at each other and smile. She knows what is coming. He holds the empty funnel upright in his hand as though it were a goblet of wine, raising it so that it dances between their faces.

"Bon appetit!" he toasts her.

There is a sound like the bleat of a goat, as gas escapes from her stomach through the tube. He is always touched by the melancholy little noise. The man tests the temperature of the eggnog with the tip of a finger, which he then licks clean.

"Just right," he says.

Now he pours from the pitcher until the topmost mark of the funnel is reached. He gives the funnel to her to hold, the way a parent will indulge a child, letting her participate. Together they watch the level in the funnel slowly fall. The woman gives a deep sigh as she feels the filling of her stomach.

"Is that good?" he asks her.

"Yes," she nods and smiles, then looks away from him, preoccupied with the feeling.

For him it is not unlike a surgical operation that has become fixed and unchanging in the hands of the man who performs it over and again. Each time there are the same instruments; the steps are followed logically; the expectation of success is high. Once it happened that the mouth of the woman suddenly filled with the eggnog. He had administered the feeding too quickly. Overdistention of the stomach had brought on reverse peristalsis, and a column of the white liquid was catapulted up toward the blocked throat with such force that the barricade of tumor was forced, and the mouth achieved. It was sudden, but he was prepared for it. With one hand, he held the curved emesis basin at her chin. With the other, he lowered the tubing to siphon the eggnog back into the funnel. In a minute the spasm was over, and the feeding was resumed. All the while that this was taking place, the man did not cease to murmur to her.

"There, there," he had said, and wiped the woman's chin with the linen napkin. Then he had waited while she struggled to control her coughing.

She had always taken pleasure in his manner toward her —a kind of gallantry that he assumed for occasions—nights when they would go to the theater, or evenings when she knew that later he would make love to her. Now, of course, she understood that his gallantry was a device. She listened to him say "lovely" and "there, there," and she tried to forget for a while what she knew too well, that at the bottom of each of these tube feedings was the sediment of despair.

It is halfway through the feeding. All at once the man is startled by the sight of something white in the bed. For a moment, he does not know what it is. In that moment of uncertainty, a line has been crossed. Then he knows that it is the eggnog running from the hole in her body, the hole from which the tube has slipped! This time, too, he understands what has happened. Just behind the inner tip of the tube, there is a little thin-walled balloon that holds just five cc. of water, enough to distend it to a size greater than that of the hole in her stomach, so that the tube will not slip out. The little balloon has broken; the tube has slipped out. Now the man gazes at the empty hole in his wife's abdomen. Despair seizes him, mounts into desperation. He knows that he must replace the old tube with a new one.

"You must do it immediately," the surgeon had warned, "or very soon, the hole will begin to shrink and heal in. Then you will not be able to insert it."

The man rises from where he has been sitting on the bed. He walks to the dresser, where the extra tube is kept. There is a hollowness in him; he hears echoes. He senses that a limit has been reached. But he clenches himself.

"It's all right," he says aloud. "Here's a new one. Don't you fret about it."

But he is sweating and his fingers tremble as he dips the end of the new tube into the pitcher of eggnog to lubricate it. Once again, he is sitting on the bed. He slides the nose of the tube into the hole. It does not go. It will not fit. So soon! Again he tries to advance the tube. It is no use. He cannot. He twists and turns it, pushing harder. The woman winces. He is hurting her! He looks up to see the knobbed purple growth bearding her face. The lopsided head she raises in her distress seems to him a strange tropical fruit, a mutant gourd that has misgrown from having been acted upon by radiation and chemicals. And so it had. It is as though he is seeing it for the first time. Once, long ago, he had gripped her neck in rage. Oh God! Did the cancer come from that? Then he remembers how he used to lap the declivities of that neck.

He pushes the tube harder. What will he do if he cannot get it in? She will starve. All at once there is a terrifying "give," and the tube slides in. He inflates the little balloon with the water he has drawn up into a syringe, injecting it into the tiny tract alongside the main channel of the thing. He pulls back on the tube until he feels it abutting against the wall of her stomach. It is done.

"There," he says.

The man rises from the bed and leaves the room. He hurries down the hall to the bathroom where he reels above the toilet and vomits with as much stealth as he can manage. In the bed, the woman hears his retching. The day before, he had brought her white peonies from the garden. He had thrust his face into the immaculate flowers and inhaled deeply. Then he had arranged them in a vase on the dresser. She gazes at them now. One of the peonies sleeps unopened, resting against the blazing wakefulness of its kin. It will not bloom, she thinks. It is a waste. For a while she had thought it might open, but not anymore. As she watches, a small breeze from the opening door sends the blind bud waving from side to side. No, she thinks. It will live asleep. To awaken would be to die.

The man returns to her bedside. He takes up the funnel to reinsert it in the tube, to resume the feeding. She reaches out and stays his hand.

"It is enough," she says. "No more."

The man flushes the tube through with a small amount of water to prevent clogging, then replaces the gauze square and the clamp.

He pulls the sheet up over her abdomen, then picks up the lacquered tray that holds the pitcher, the napkin ring, the emesis basin, and the white enamel funnel. At the door he turns and smiles.

"You take a nice little nap, now," he says.

Her eyes are already closed.

In the kitchen, the man washes the pitcher and the funnel, and, climbing on a chair, he puts them away on the top shelf of the cupboard. At the rear, where he won't be apt to see them again for a long time.

THE MIRROR: A TALE OF ARAN

BITTER AND FELL is winter in the islands of Aran. All night the cold sharpens itself on the rasp of the wind, and by dawn is gone so hard there is nothing more it can do, nowhere else it can go but into burning. So that the line between heat and cold is muddled, and one feels a fierce silver bead in the chest. Underneath the breastbone cringes the heart. There is an island called Inishmar that is the smallest of those that are inhabited. Inishmar has not the consolation of trees. The only soil has been scraped from here and there, shovel by hard shovel, and packed into holes and sheltered gulleys. Such islands are like insects that long ago were shaken off in annoyance by the great masses of land and ever since lie shiny and helpless at some decent remove from the back of the earth.

Once upon a time, not so long ago as to be forgotten, nor so recently as to be part of this time, an old man and an old woman lived on the island. It seemed they had always been there, and except for once, neither had left it. When the old man was a boy of seven years, there had been a winter harsher than ever before. Not for a minute did the murderous sea lighten or cease to slide back and forth across all but the very highest part of the rock, where the cottage stood. They had run out of food, and he had begun to cough. His mother blamed it on the fairies who had vexed her all her life and would not let up, she said, until they had pestered her to death. In the autumn, she had dug her potatoes and found that one had been scooped out and filled with blood. And now there was this wild winter. They had run out of food altogether, and the boy had gotten a bad chest. It was the fairies all right, she said.

Ye've got to go, the boy heard her say to his father, and take the boy to Ireland. A moment later, without waiting for his answer, she said, Well go then, and that was all. He remembered being lifted into the curragh, and the hellish rowing of the man. How his father gripped the oars so that man and wood seemed to have fused. And he remembered the terrible groans that came from his father's mouth, that were gathered from somewhere in his back and flung to the wind. They frightened him, these loud passionate sounds. All the more because he could not marry them to the man who often spent an entire day without speech. He could not remember his father's face, only the whiteness of it, and the way his beard blew over one shoulder. When they reached Ireland, his father had pulled the boat up on the beach, and died. Just toppled back into the boat. Heartburst, he had heard the men say. The next day they had taken him back. There were two curraghs this time. In one was his father and three men. He was in the other with three more. He had never been away from Inishmar since then.

The men of Ireland had carried the body of his father to the hut, and showed it to his mother. They asked her where it was to be buried, for there seemed to them no plot of ground large enough on this rock. She led them to a place nearby, which was a basin in the stone, molded by the curling of the seas that washed over the top and back again. Sand and earth and bits of shell and seaweed had been gathered here and packed in this place which was for them a garden. Here, she said, put him here.

And the men had measured out the size of the grave with sticks, leaving just an inch to spare, for they knew the cost of the ground to this woman and her child. And there they dug, scooping out the meager soil with great care. The boy had never seen so much earth laid bare, and to him it was like the sight of jewels. And then their shovels struck something hard. Ah, said one of the men, it is too shallow here. But they dug farther to lay bare the rock, and saw that it was no rock but something white and smooth. And when his mother saw it, she knelt by the side of the grave and reached in and drew out the skull of her own mother, for it was just here, in this place, that they had laid her long ago. And the boy watched her where she had howled then, this woman who had not yet wept, but whose grief had been set in motion by the touch of her mother's skull. In the end, the men laid them in together, covered them up and tamped it down. Then they went into their curraghs and they rowed away.

Now it was sixty years later and a fierce winter again. The old man and the old woman had never felt so bad a time. There was food enough for but a few more days. Soon they would be too weak to keep the fire going. When it went out, they would die. Days went by, and they did not speak to each other, for each feared that any words would let loose the dread they had been holding in. At last, she saw him go to the box where the few coins were. He tied them into a piece of cloth and put it inside his shirt. Then, he walked to the door, silent until his hand was lifting the very latch itself, holding out still against the words, fearing the magical effect they would surely have, and the old woman felt helpless with her unshuttered ears.

"I'll have to be going now," he said.

His voice startled her. She had not heard him speak in three days, and it sounded alien to her, like the noise of an animal that had somehow come to a place which was not its native habitat. Perhaps it had ridden there on an iceberg, or been blown to it on the wind, and now that she heard its cry, the sound made her shiver with fright, the way she did when she heard the fairies bark and giggle in the corners.

"Well, go then," she said after a long time. And they both understood that the time of horror was upon them.

The old woman stood in the doorway and watched him climb down to the wet rocks. They were alternately silvery with the foam of the waves, and black with the wetness left behind. She watched him heft the curragh to his back. His head was hidden by it, so that all she could see of him were his sticklike legs and that boat shell that he wore like a beetle. Now he was standing in the sea holding the curragh in front of him, waiting for an opening in the waves so that he could race between them and slam the curragh down for just time enough to jump in and keep it from swamping. She had seen him do it many times before, but now it seemed to her impossible to do, and that in a while he would back out of the sea, set down the curragh, and climb back up to her so that they could just let it go, give it up. At the last minute, she decided that was what she had wanted all along, and she almost started to run down to the rocks to call out to him to come back, to stop. But she did not, could not. Not after all the silence. And a shyness came over the old woman, and she stayed in the doorway watching him as though he were a strange man that she had watched every day and wanted to speak to but could not.

Then she saw him take a running step and fall forward into the boat with his hands gripping the gunwales on either side, balancing the curragh somehow while it scooped wildly. In a minute he had the oars unshipped, was sitting there, pulling. And with each pull, getting smaller until he was just a speck in her eye, a speck which she wiped away with one finger, after which she turned and went back into the cottage and closed the door. The old woman bent to stir the turf in the fire, then sat down to wait.

It was bad luck to let a fire go out. Someone always died, or the roof fell in, or the fairies came and poisoned the potatoes with their urine. Most of her life, the old woman had picked at the fire, separating bits of turf, then heaping them together, turning them over this way and that. For her, keeping fire on this island all surrounded and washed with water was a victory of some kind, and, like all triumphs, had taken upon itself certain magic properties. Only once, the fire had gone out. In the middle of the night, she had awakened with a terrible choking in her chest. She could not catch her breath, and sat up to find that the fire had gone out. Then she had heard a dog wailing, and the next day she had dug her potatoes and found that one had been filled with blood. The fairies would never lose a chance like that.

All that day the old man rowed, bending, straightening, then doubling again in the rhythm pounded out for him by the thumping of the sea against the bottom of the curragh. The sounds that came from his throat with each pull were the grunts of a body laboring to be delivered of something impacted deep inside. His lips and eyes burned; his beard, which in the beginning rose and fell with his body, now lay still, pulled to one shoulder, and frozen there, fused to the ice of his shoulder.

It was toward dusk. Already the first stars were dividing up the sky. In an hour there would be no more sight, only hearing. On and on he rowed, an ancient machine that would soon run down when its momentum was spent. Dimly, he saw a gull stooping to the waves. All at once, the man felt a strange uncertainty of his flesh, as though it were pausing for a moment, confused, wondering which way to fall, then deciding at last that toward the oars would be best. He tumbled upon them, swiveling back and forth with the energy with which he had infused them. Now that he was through, they had enough to go on without him, and they did—or so it seemed to the old man, cradled and waiting to die.

When the shout came, the shout that was not a bird, nor a false construction of wind and wave, but a sound from the mouth of a fellow human being, he did not move. Who can trust the hailing from the shadowy banks of such a river? It was better to lie rocking, with the eyes closed.

More shouting. The old man smiled, floated. When the hands gripped his shoulders, tipped him backward, he was ready to be taken, offered his breast. He would not resist. And they seized him! And lifted him, and carried him to where there was no motion but a solid hard place that he recognized as . . . the Earth. The old man was sorrowful then, as though something—a prize—for which he had labored with all his might had been denied him at the last minute. All that rowing, that cold, that sea. He opened his eyes and saw the sky infected with gray, felt the cold spray, touched stones at his fingertips. He had rowed all the way to Ireland! The way his father had done. And with that thought came a landslide of coughs and retching, the gasps that made him feel a fish disenfranchised from the sea.

When he awoke, he knew that he had eaten. He was warm and dry. They told him that it was two days since he had come. Later, he rose and walked to the sea. It was calm as death. He thought, now it is time to go back. The old woman was waiting for him. The men of Ireland put the grain and potatoes into the curragh and lifted it into the water, held it while he climbed in and took hold of the oars. They pushed him off. He was in the sea again.

But now something burned against the skin of his chest, beneath his sweaters and coat. He felt it and smiled and did not mind the pain in his joints as he pulled the oars. For he had narrowed all his senses down to that one spot on the left side of his chest over the ribs, near the heart. It was what the old man had stolen—he who had never stolen before. From whom should he steal? The old woman?

In Ireland one night, he had awakened on the mat they had laid for him by the fire. The others lay sleeping nearby. He had gotten up to go outside to relieve himself. When he returned, he saw upon a shelf a piece of glass encased in a thin wooden frame with a handle attached. He had picked it up, brought it to the fire, and looked at it, then *in* it, and had seen there a face—a terrible old face—like a wild man's, whose sunken eyes were blue as fairy-flax, with a tempest of white hair, and lips caked with something dark that had gathered in the corners of the mouth and dried there. Terrible as it was, something held him to it, perhaps the answering stare of him who was trapped there within the glass. And soon a recollection gathered, faint and dim, from his childhood, something he did not know the name of. He saw the awakening, the wild surmise grow in the face of the man in the glass as well. At last the old man brought the mirror closer to his face, straining, reaching out for whatever it was that was coming near to him after so many years, and then, with the glass touching his lips, he heard his own voice whisper, "Da . . . Da."

And the sound of the word was like the hissing of fire, for he saw the lips of the other one form the very word he had whispered. Then he knew that trapped within that glass was the father who had rowed all the way to Ireland so long ago, and whom he had thought to have died, whom he had seen buried, but who was somehow living and imprisoned in the bit of glass! He knew also that he would have that bit of glass, would steal it, must. There would be this rescue. He had been saved for it. And he, who had never stolen, became sly. He slipped the glass beneath his shirt, and lay back upon the mat, feeling the part of him it touched shiver and burn, as hot and bright as the sun.

Now in the curragh, the old man felt strangely aroused. It was an agitation. Sudden sweat broke from his papery skin. A fine trembling took his chest. But they were more the symptoms of an acute illness than the effects of the charge that he, all at once, understood had been laid upon him. By whom? He did not know, only that he had come through his ordeal and had made a discovery, had found the surprise at the very center of his life, and that it had changed him. He would never be the same as he was.

For the old man, the rowing home was an escape, a getting away, and, as such, was done with that remarkable ease with which superhuman feats are accomplished by men who are goaded by fire, or placed in combat with ferocious beasts. A new juice flows; there is a numbness wherein pain is not felt, nor fear realized. In just such a state of blind vigor, the old man rowed across the sea. It was an act of rescue. And, all the while, he felt the mirror against his chest as though it were a mouth applied there, through which energy surged from some mysterious source into his body, flooding it, galvanizing his stiff joints, his stringy muscles, moistening and lubricating him until he was once again a working machine.

Somewhere in that time of bending and straightening, he thought, I'll not show it to her. "No," he said aloud, "no, it is mine." And although the words were ripped from his lips by the wind so that the old man did not hear the sound of his voice, they were as irrevocable as the thought that produced them.

At last the old man pulled the curragh out of the water

and secured it upon the high rocks of Inishmar. Inside the hut, the old woman was bending at the fire, stirring it. She looked up to see him, and gladness came over her. "So you are back," she said, and continued to stir the fire. She knew without asking what he had endured, all the rigor of it. He carried the sacks from the curragh to the hut, and she stored them, marking her efforts with little grunts and whispers.

That night, as the old woman lay asleep, he rose from his pallet, and stepped to the far side of the chimney. There he gouged with his knife into the hardened mud that was the caulking between the stones until he had loosened a large one, level with his head. Slowly then, he drew it out, and, in the little space behind, he placed the mirror. He put back the stone, and returned to his bed. Each day when the old woman left the hut to gather seaweed from the rocks for drying, he would go to the fireplace, slide out the stone, and hold up the mirror to the light. "Da," he said over and over, and he would see his father's face take on that soft gaze of love for which he had yearned all of his life. When he saw the old woman approaching the door, he would quickly replace the mirror and the stone and walk away.

Weeks passed, and one day as he was looking into the mirror, he saw that she had come back, and was standing in the doorway. "What have you?" she said. "It is nothing," he said. "A bit of stone." And he hid it in his hand. But the old woman had seen. And she stalked him, until one night, as she pretended to lie asleep, she saw him rise from his bed and go to the fireplace, saw him take out the *thing* which now she must see. She watched him hold it over the open fire and gaze at it, and saw how his face grew tender and soft, and all at once she knew that it was the picture of a young, beautiful girl that he had met in Ireland, and with whom he had fallen in love. And for the first time she sensed the horror of her life on the island, Inishmar, that had become for her the image of her mind. She saw herself as bald, barren, a boulder against which the sea crashed, and whose buffeting she had not felt until that moment.

Now! She watched him, waiting for his sleep, anticipating it with more excitement than she thought still danced in her nerves. At last, she saw that letting go, that small collapse that told her that the old man slept. In the hazy light of the turf fire, his face seemed made of plaster upon which crept, now here, now there, a gray mold. And she thought of a corpse she had seen years ago rolling in the sea, crashing again and again upon the rocks. She remembered how oblivious it was to the banging, how its solemn expression never changed. For a brief moment, she was swept by a kind of sorrow for the old man, and she remembered how once he had been as cool and fresh as a seagull. She lay back upon her pallet, then. But when she could no longer see his face, she thought of what he had done, how he was cheating her of something. And her rage blazed, for she fed it with an image of soft golden hair and smooth breasts and cheeks.

She stood then, looking down at him. At that moment, there was more life in her than she could sustain. She was afraid that she might fall down and die of it then and there. But that she could not do, not until she had seen the picture. At the side of the fireplace, she felt blindly, ran her flapping fingers over the stones until she found the loose one. Then scrabbling, rocking, pulling and scraping, she edged it out. How heavy it was! It fell back against her chest, where she clutched it tightly. The old woman lowered the stone to the hearth with utmost daintiness. She reached into the space. Yes! It was there, that thing that was only his, and not hers, and that she had to see even though she knew it would kill her to see it. Once she had it in her hand, she grew calm, as though its hardness were given over somehow to her flesh. She stopped her trembling. She could no longer feel the pressure of her heartbeat against her jaw.

Suddenly, the old man groaned in his sleep, and raised his thin arms as though to ward off a bad dream. She waited for him to go still again, then knelt upon the hearth and leaned as far as she could into the firelight. The old woman held up the mirror . . . and recoiled. This was no beautiful young girl, but an ugly old hag! With a drooping nose over thin gray lips and a bundle of dead hair. A thousand wrinkles carved up this horror. It was the ugliest face she had ever seen. A witch, she thought, a horrible witch, and shuddering with disgust, she watched the face in the mirror draw back its lips in a grimace. All at once, her whole body felt as though it were being squeezed into a place that was too small for it, and raising her arm high above her head, the old woman threw the mirror against the hearthstones with all her might.

The noise of the shattering woke the old man, and he spoke into the darkness, without turning to see, "What is it?"

"Nothing," said the old woman. "Nothing at all. It's the fairies have been and gone."

THE SPECIMEN COLLECTORS

THERE IS A little-known race of men about which I feel it my duty to warn the general public. They are called pathologists. These men present to the world as their high purpose the diagnosis of disease based on the laboratory examination of either all (*O terrore!*) or some portion of the body, their materials having been excavated in their morgues or snipped off for them by only slightly less scurrilous surgeons. Such is the livelihood of pathologists. But what of their passion? And dark it is, rapacious. For these are the dreadful Specimen Collectors of Medicine. Cynical, jaded men who scorn your workaday carrion, and pant only after corporeal exotica much as the gourmet who despises porridge but would sell his father's name for a ragout of cuckoo tongue. So unscrupulous they, that not even the liver of Saint Sebastian would be outside their traffic, but the Dear Piece must be snatched from its reliquary to turn up a year later in Bratislava, say, dried and pinned to a cork board on the wall of some godless Czech pathologist. Beneath it, doubtless, some shameless legend: "Liver of saint with stellate laceration, anterior surface, right lobe. Unusually good condition." A casual lunch with two pathologists is likely to reveal that one owns a piece of an early Christian, the other the rear footpad of a lion.

Behold the specimen collector at work. The great stone morgue is alive with activity. It is a very Baghdad bazaar.

Beneath the fluorescent lights, on a dozen slabs, lies the "catch" in various stages of evisceration and dismemberment. Each corpse wears upon its great toe a label bearing its name. A "twisty" is used to secure it there. It is said that the mere act of dying seems to confer upon all of us the appearance of beatitude, as though each one has been freshly taken down from the Cross. In the morgue, this is not believable.

Step aside! A gurney rattles in, bringing a newcomer. Now another gurney evacuates a graduate toward the hearse gaping at the end of a ramp. Interns, residents, dieners and licensed embalmers, each wearing a long gray lab coat, tug, haul, and slice, all the while calling out to each other in hearty voice. Their brains seem but feebly illuminated, like those of men who pass sentence or carry out execution. What clatter of cutlery! What rivers of multicolored water! One knows at once that here, at least, the world's work is being done.

Above each of the slabs, there is a hanging scale such as is used in delicatessen stores. Now and then, a kidney will flop up on the scale, then bounce itself to stillness. "Right kidney . . . 200 grams," a voice calls out. Somewhere this is recorded. The kidney is retrieved from the scale; cubes and slices of it are taken and arranged on trays. From these pieces, microscopic slides will be made.

In the morgue, then, a great tussling herd, heads and rumps rising, falling. And everywhere a clanging, a jostling, a shouting. Into this clamor slouches the dread pathologist. He wears the grayest lab coat of all. He sidles along the awful avenues between the slabs, deaf to the greetings of the others. His neck is wry; his mouth hangs open, the lips moist, the tongue lolling between. How quickly he scuttles! It is no wonder. Word has reached him that one of the bodies, a woman, harbors in her left ovary a dermoid cyst containing three perfectly formed teeth, two molars and a canine. He will, he *must* have it, and hastens toward his prize as glinty as a streetwalker stepping up to a sailor. In a moment he is at her, rummaging; his shoulders hunch; his elbows are furious. Now and then, he turns his head to shoot a glance behind him, the way a pigeon will do, standing guard over a potato chip. Minutes later, he straightens. Something round and pink is in his hand. It is not a peach.

No, gentle reader, pathology is not the most delicate of the medical arts. I have known a pathologist who, armed with a tree trunk and a couple of paving stones, could pass for Cyclops. This same man has been observed playing "soldier" with a collection of lithopedions that he keeps in a cigar box in a locked drawer. These "stone babies" are the calcified result of pregnancies which, by one route or another, have found their way into the free peritoneal cavity. In that he causes no symptoms, the innocent little lithopedion is discovered by purest chance. Surgeons in search of other, more dangerous game, will come upon him in the environs of some organ beneath which, slumbrous, he has lain for many years, and from which den he never thought to leave. He, whose gentle fate was to have kept everlasting watch among the bones and the dust of his mother, is now untimely pluck'd and delivered into the world as statuary. His sleepless permanence now disturbed, he shall like Ozymandias, King of Kings, crumble into sand.

The best place to see a pathologist is in the basement of a medical school. There, where the walls sweat and trickle, where whispers echo through uncarpeted tunnels, and where great pipes course along the ceiling carrying God-knows-what effluent from the premises. Among these dews and damps, he nethers, shouldering from tank to slab and back again, his eyes hooded, and always in hand a bottle or tray the contents of which are best left unspecified. Where he passes, a chill gathers; you catch the rank whiff of formaldehyde. Should such a man smile at you, be on guard. His grin may be no impulse toward congeniality but a crafty device to lay hold of some part of you upon which his acquisitive eye has fastened.

Just as pets are said to take on some of the physical features of their masters, so does the pathologist each year grow more whey-faced and thin, so does he fall into long silences, so does he become more reminiscent of the material with which he works. Of what does such a man dream? In the unsoiled regions of sleep do beautiful women come to him, smiling? Do they feed him cold grapes in bannered pavilions? Or is it some ulcered stomach that he sees just beyond his grasp, toward which a hated rival races? I have often suspected that some hideous and secret covenant lay behind this fanatical accumulation of human flesh. These grim suspicions are not easily proven, since the perpetrators are a canny tribe, all of whom have closed their mouths on the pill of silence. As soon ask a horse why he eats fodder.

Enter the subterranean study of a pathologist, and you are in the cave of Grendel. From the ceiling, suspended by wires, hang lungs, the delicate arborizations of which are filled with red, white, and blue rubber; red for the arteries, blue for the veins, and the bronchial tree done in white, all conspiring to the illusion of a garden of patriotic blooms. As the door clicks gassily shut behind you, the lungs are set in motion by the breeze. You look about. At first there is no sign of life. All is silent, still. Suddenly, you hear a cough! Terrified, you stare at the swinging lungs. Could it be! Now something scurries! A segment of the offal strewn upon the floor stirs, lifts, and arranges itself into the shape of a human being. You blink, and there he hunkers, sorting bones, one of which suggests a recent severe gnawing. The very idea of all those bones! From God-knows-how-many unrelated corpses pitted and brought to conclave by no last wish of their living owners, but by the unslakable thirst of the specimen collector. Gone, any hoped-for corporeal integrity; gone, eternal solitude. A man ought to have the comfort of knowing that he will either lie alone in splendor, or next to his most congenial companion. But higgledy-piggledy your skull, my pelvis? No offense, but, well, I'd prefer not to. Our said parts having achieved no such propinquity in life, I see no reason why they should be thrust together clackety-clack in death. In the office of the pathologist, except for the organs of the great and near great, all of the specimens are anonymous. It seems a soulless thing to cut out the best part of a man, and fail to label it: Liver of Henry Huckaby, b. 1914, d. 1977. It is little enough to do. Perhaps a droll or goodnatured epitaph would do. Something like:

Saving This Piece, May the Rest Rest in Peace.

If for no other reason than to preserve the integrity of your remains from pathologists, immediate cremation would seem the only possible choice of a decorous man. In the words of Thomas Browne,

To be gnaw'd out of our graves, to have our sculs made drinking bowls, and our bones turned into pipes to delight and sport our Enemies, are Tragicall abominations, escaped in burning Burials.

I am firmly of the belief that pathologists are born and not made. I have observed even first-year interns hurrying from the morgue to their lockers with some bit of finger, the odd kneecap. It is a thought that saddens the heart. If these things be done in the green tree, what shall be done in the dry? And pathologists go it alone. They have forgone the banter and slap of fellowship, preferring their private, more recondite joys. Perhaps I should be kinder. Perhaps they are the victims of the slow toxin of formaldehyde that produces a chemical madness; perhaps they have heard too long the nightingale of Death caroling in their drafty halls, and have become enchanted at the sound, ever after to be ruled by a wild taste. Is the pathologist then so different from the poet, the composer or painter who strives to solidify into art his secret delight? For each man, his own poetry; although some, written in runic rhyme, is indecipherable by the rest of us. It is quite to be expected that the specimen collector would issue it in his will that he be buried with full Pathological Honors—in Lung and Monstrosity—Thus, up to his neck in pickled treasure, he would disdain the death that for others holds out such fear.

The truth is that pathology is less an occupation concerned with diagnosis, than a preoccupation with the oddments and endments of the flesh. So famished are its practitioners for specimens that, in time, they become themselves a confusion of hungers. Hence their reprehensible penchant for comparing the manifestations of disease to items of food. As in "cheesy pus," "coffee-ground vomitus," "nutmeg liver," "currant jelly stool," and the *peau d'orange* breast of cancer. In this, they have the precedent of Petronius who likened the perianal warts of his boy-lovers unto an "orchard of figs." Let a pathologist read aloud his reports, and every decent gorge rises. Tumors are the size of grapes, walnuts, plums, eggs, lemons, oranges, grapefruit, and melons. Pumpkin and watermelon being invoked only for the rare ovarian cyst. And while it is not, strictly speaking, one of the edibilia, toothpaste is the favorite simile for the stools passed in obstructive jaundice. Toothpaste and stool! A sophomoric misalliance indeed.

It is in the nature of pathologists that they are easily provoked to rage and violence. I have known one so fastidious as to require three bites in the eating of a single cherry. This same man could bare-handle a brain out of its skull in something under three minutes from first incision to the reefing up. Another, who was rendered dyspneic by a minuet, would hew at a cow, root and branch, to wrest from it a tiny trophy of pituitary. And I recall one pathologist on the faculty of the medical school that I attended. His prize possession was a cyclops, a one-eyed full-term monstrosity that sported a tubular proboscis. The thing swam in a great sealed jar of formaldehyde on his desk. Rumor had it that Professor Fenstermacher sang German lullabies to it in the dead of night. One day, the cyclops, jar and all, was missing from his desk. To this day I shudder at the image of him stalking the aisles of the laboratory where we students shrank over our microscopes. In his hand, a huge femur which he waved about like a cudgel.

"Tsyklops," he strangled, "he iss gone. Somevun hass taken my Tsyklops. Vich vun off you hass taken my Tsyklops from me?" He would surely have laid out any number of us with his femur had not a gifted ventriloquist in our midst called out:

"Schwartzkopf!"

At the sound of the name of his most hated rival, Fenstermacher froze, his eyes silver slits of murder.

"Jawohl! Schwartzkopf!" he nickered, and, brandishing the bone like a troll, he lurched from the room. Later, a substitute was called in to teach the class for the duration of his sentence.

Such specimen collectors are medical mutineers who see flesh as art deco rather than as the spirit thickened. Now what is the time-honored method of dealing with mutineers? Why, they are brought before a tribunal of officers and peers, convicted, and shot through the heart by their shipmates. For these latter know well that a mutinous mind is a weevil in a sack of flour. It must be extracted for the greater good of society.

So would I exhort all honest internists, pediatricians, and family practitioners to drive the swine of pathology from the temple of Aesculapius, and herd them into some apt enclosure where they can be picked off with a minimum of mess.

TRAVELS IN RHINELAND

WHAT IS LIKE unto the tongue, O Lord? What is like unto the tongue?

Dewy flap; goalie to the throat, cheek-char; mop-gum; a muscle from whose trembly tip poetry drips, like saliva. Watch a dog pumping at his dish, a cat, precise at a fish head, and know the cunning of the tongue. Who has not felt his bones melt when he hears from the next room a tongue crooning to itself? Or watched snow falling on the outthrust tongue of a child? They say a man grows old when he begins to hide his tongue, entombing it in his mouth. But, the tongue of an old man is sweetened by the memory of its travels.

No matter its report in decibels, whether hushed, smacking or pistol shot, a kiss is but a kiss until the nimble tongue, like Eden's fabled snake, insinuates among the quartet of lips foregathered. Then is the whole calm congress transported to violent Paradise. So browse away, Tongue, thou groom and cradle of love. For such work, a thousand of you would not surfeit be.

The ancients put a divine gloss on things. In their prayers, the Egyptians exhorted Pharaoh to use his tongue as the steering pole of the boat of Maat, the god of trust. Another Egyptian god, Bes, had a protruding tongue that he used to protect against evil spirits during childbirth. Bes

186

is also the bestower of jollity, and the surveillant of music. (Lovely god!) According to the Indian myth of creation, the god Bhim pulled out his tongue, stretching it "out and out until it was a road fit for carts to travel from the underworld to the sky." The hanging tongue has long since lost its religious significance, replaced, I suppose, by the hanging pendant or lavaliere. Artistically, the tongue is now seen only in happy puppets.

Stick out your tongue! Now put it away! Legion are the tongues which advance or retreat at the command of a doctor. By such generalship does he come to discover and conquer whole provinces of disease. Is the tongue beefy and red? Is it pale? Swollen? Fissured? Coated with a brown and hairy residue? Does it reek? Glow in the dark? Is it yellow on the underside? Skewed to the right or left? Just as the scout places his ear to the ground to hear the transmission of distant hoofbeats, so does the doctor fix his gaze upon the telltale tongue for signs of trouble far away.

The human tongue is a dense mat of interlacing muscle fibers which cross and recross it from front to back and from side to side in infinite combination. These *intrinsic* muscles are in addition to the *extrinsic* muscles which root the tongue to the floor of the mouth and the pharynx. All together, they work to flatten, broaden, shorten, retract, curl, and bulge the tongue; to depress it at the tip, or in the middle in order to make a concavity to receive food; to protrude, elevate, draw forward and upward, downward and backward. The tongue cannot, however, slither from the mouth to sun itself upon a rock, or lash off on a little airing. In this, it is hindered by its thick root. Still, like the tree, which arborizes fantastically and bursts into bloom, so does the hobbled tongue spill its voice into the air. All of earshot is its domain.

Working in harmony with the palates (soft and hard), the teeth, lips, cheek, mandible, and pharyngeal wall, the tongue articulates sound. To change its position in the resonating chamber of the mouth is to alter the tone of a sound. When the tongue abuts against the gums, teeth, and palate, the friction and plosion of consonant speech is produced. Still, for some consonants, the tongue simply lies down dumb on the floor of the mouth, letting the bullets fly overhead. As in p, b, m, f, and h. Just so did the well-hung tongues of Cicero and Caruso elevate the spirit of man.

It is to the muscular structure of the tongue that we owe the management of food once it has passed the threshold of the lips. The mouthful is rolled to the occluding surfaces of the teeth, crushed against the hard palate and mixed with saliva to make a swallowable mash. Later, the remnants of the meal are swept from the teeth by the tongue, for which role the roughness of its dorsal surface is well suited, preventing as it does slippage and slidage. This roughness is more pronounced in herbivorous beasts and ruminants, which makes one wonder whether the elimination of meat from the diet would accentuate this feature in man. If so, one were well advised to ruminate before taking a vegetarian lover. A simple tongue depressor and flashlight at the plighting might avoid a lifetime of painful abrasions. Only after its janitorial work is done is the honest tongue content to wallow in its salivary fastness, memorializing banquets.

These and other glories of the tongue notwithstanding, it is the nose that arouses my own deepest passions. Oh, let me at last confess it! I am a . . . yes . . . a nasophiliac. Let others dream of bosoms, napes, toes, what have you. Only give me a nose. To feel upon my neck its humid breeze, watch the ruffle of translucent nose wings, see its small shadow cast across the vermilion border of the lip, that is to me very heaven.

It all began at the age of twelve, while gazing at a painting of Saint George and the Dragon. Ah, the ineffable power of art.

Behold! The molten monster squats,
Grenade! Upon the steaming rocks.

But it is the snout that captures. Nostrils dark and wide enough to nest a family of wrens. From these nose-holes—salvos. They burst above the shell-pink maiden, who turns her gaze upon the beast with that sweetest of confusions—terror and desire.

Enter Saint George in full metallic fig. He is shamelessly noble. In one hand he holds a sword, a shield in the other. In aim most murderous, his arm is raised above the coiled beast. Whilst, stirred by the currents of the battle, a single length of opaque gauze flutters between the maiden's thighs, and billows up to hide her nipples, the artist having managed to show her stark naked and fully clothed at one and the same time.

Show me a youth who would not burn to go in liege to that knight as Rescuer's Assistant, show me such an one, and I will show you a boy deficient in hormones. Set Honor in one eye, and Lust in his other, and he shall go the scarlet every time. But, slay the dragon! The very thought is obscene. Slay the dragon! For doing everything I always wanted to do but didn't have the nose for? Never. My sympathies were all with the dragon. And so began my life of nasophilia.

More than any other part, it is the nose that *presents*. It is the triumphal arch under which the other organs lie low and unobtrusive. Beneath this eminence must every smallest bit of food pass on its way to the stomach, pausing for a moment to pay obeisance. Through it is blown the breath of life, warmed and filtered. Here, each scent is told, be it reek or attar. And the nose is Cerberus guarding the lungs, trapping particulate matter in its hair and mucus, lest dirt be swept in, and harm be done.

As to olfaction, it is the most ancient of the senses, yet the least well understood. The fact is that you do not know how you smell. Nor what it is that makes an onion smell the way it does, nor exactly how that property reaches the brain of the smeller. The whole process is mysterious, curtained from us, and given over to outlandish hypothesis. We smell, and that, apparently, is that.

Still let us try:

In man, the olfactory cells cover but one single square inch of the body, part of which is on the outer wall of each nasal passage, and part on the nasal septum. Each olfactory cell is a tiny rod with a knob at its more superficial end. From this knob, a fine filament of hair protrudes into a sea of mucus. Without this mucus, we could not trap the droplets of odor. For any odor is no more than a cloud of tiny droplets emanating from a moist surface, and dispersed therefrom. The odorant is transferred from the mucus to the little hair, to the olfactory cell to a fine nerve fiber that emerges from the narrower end. This nerve fiber goes to join many others to make up the olfactory nerve which winds upward to the olfactory lobes of the brain. As with all the machinery of the body, the apparatus of olfaction works more finely for some than for others. Certain of us smell almost nothing at all and would be quite at ease in the must and fust of the Orient. Still others think of, say, Korea, impacted with night soil and kimchi, as a huge closet in which something awful lies bloating. It is regretable that with the ascendancy of sight and hearing, and the gift of intelligence, man has forgotten how to smell, and this atrophied sense is constricted now to matters of wine and eau de cologne.

To some "olfactory sensitives," the least soupçon of fetor or fragrance is apparent. Among the people bearing such a "dog's nose" are those remarkable folk who, suffering from a strange confusion of their senses, are able to smell blue and yellow. One such "olfactory sensitive" was Saint Catherine of Siena, who was forever remarking on the overpowering smell of blood. This was most dramatically recounted in a letter to her confessor Fra Raimondo da Capua in which she told of being present at the beheading of a young nobleman wrongly accused of treason. She had successfully converted him just prior to his execution. In order to sustain his faith, she determined to accompany the youth to the moment of his death. Kneeling in front of the block, she held the youth's head until, with the thunk of the axe, it came free in her arms. It was then that she smelled the blood. "When he was at rest my soul rested in peace and quiet, and in so great fragrance of blood that I could not bear to remove the blood which had fallen on me from him." Now, I have been around a lot of blood in my life. Whole days and nights have seen me, neck and toe, imbrued with gore. Nor have I detected the least niff, the smallest whiff to emanate from it in the freshly shed state. Did Catherine own a dog's nose which finds nothing in the natural world devoid of odor? Or am I to add to my already depressing list of declining powers sanguinary anosmia?

Scent and sainthood do seem to have had a more than customary relationship. Saint Joseph of Copertino was able to recognize the sins of the flesh by their odor, a talent that would not wear very well with friends and neighbors. Both Saint Paconi and Saint Philip Neri would gag at the smell of heretics. When the grave of Saint Thomas à Becket was opened, those present were rendered faint by the delicious fragrance. And after the death of Saint Theresa, a saltcellar which had been placed on her bed retained a wonderful odor. The pus of Saint John of the Cross was truly laudable in that it was redolent of lilies. To the skeptic who would suggest that this was due to diabetes or an infection with Pseudomonas aeruginosa, I say, *tant pis pour vous!* This is not to say that all saintly odors were good. The odor diffused around his pillar by Saint Simeon Stylites can hardly be called sweet. Still, some people do smell naturally good. All babies do, and, according to Plutarch, Alexander the Great, whose tunic seemed to have been soaked in perfume. Why, even Walt Whitman is reported to have smelled good!

In matters of smell it is *chacun à son gout*. A man will be prone to loud outrage at the passage of another's flatus, yet be oddly pleased by his own. It is a peasant wisdom that informs that each man loves the smell of his own farts. It is further evidence of Heaven's munificence that unrepelled by our own stink, we do not smell ourselves as others smell us. That which is sulfurous and putrescent to another is lilied waftage to the one who is to the odor born. Gardyloo, gardyloo, cried the scullions of eighteenth century Edinburgh only seconds before they flung their slops and swipes from the window to the street below. A safe two centuries later, we dab our nostrils with eau de cologne, and we shudder. He that invites me to dine on gorgonzola sets a table too high for me. Such a man would play with skunks, and only a severe shunning by his companions would awaken him to his ill-odor.

One tastes only on contact; one can smell at a distance. So powerful is the odor of vanillin that it is perceptible at 0.000000005 gram per liter of air. A breath of smoke and you run in time to escape from your burning house. You smell bacon or freshly baked bread, and your saliva flows, your gastric juice is liberated. You smell putrid meat, and you are warned away; you lose your appetite. The nose is truly the sentinel to the body.

But mere admiration of the nose of man grows into worship when one considers the olfactory talents of the other creatures. Hero's summoning of Leander from across the Dardanelles was nothing compared to the attractiveness of a moth shedding pheromones into the air. Insectivorous plants lure flies to their death by exuding a smell like that of rotten meat. And the ant finds his way home by smell alone. Paint the eyes of an ant with opaque varnish, and you will "embarrass" him; amputate his antennae, the site of his olfactory cells, and he will go hopelessly astray. Does the ant map out a field of odor in his travels, and then merely retrace the chemical topography in order to reach home?

The far-flung summons of an odor sends a dog rollicking off through the woods. Still, were one harnessed with the olfactory sense of a dog, a simple walk around the block would surely lead to madness and death what with squirrels, garbage, other dogs, cats, and assorted excremental goodies. Let man be consoled in that, of all creatures (*pace* Ferdinand the Bull), he alone smells for the pleasure of it. In this does he approach the gods.

Despite that smell is our most ancient sense, odors remain nameless. Does it matter? A rose by any name . . . still smells. But it is true that language owns no words for smells as it does for colors, touch, sounds. *Faute de mieux*, we pin a smell to what it smells like, as in *goatish* or *garlicky*, *feculent* or *ammoniacal*. Or we plunder the vocabulary of taste to call an odor *sweet* or *sour*. Even, we invoke the effect that an odor produces, as in *nauseating* or *sickening*. Words like *dank* and *stuffy* are general, too inconclusive, whilst *mephitic* has lost its importance since brimstone stopped being mentioned in sermons. And *mawkish?* Well, just what do maggots smell like? Perhaps man was not meant to name this most primitive of his powers. Perhaps there awaits for the rash poke-nose who dares defy the god of olfaction, a retributive anosmia. For one so arrogant, might not all the world's smells be suddenly canceled? A thousand times rather would I dwell in the stinkdom of goats, awash with their hircine fetor than ride blandly through a world of odorlessness, minus the bouquet of a rose. Good Lord! In such a world, the distinction between white wine and urine would depend on taste! Therefore, let us hush and make obeisance.

Aristotle made the assumption that good-smelling things are good for you, and bad-smelling things bad. This has not always been the case, not in medicine or religion at least. Remember that burning hair and feathers is done to drive out demons, and that sulphur was burned in the streets during plagues. There are those of us who find the aroma of smoldering tobacco rather pleasant, but the sight of a doctor smoking a cigarette is enough to roil the intestine of his least righteous colleague. It would seem that a man who has sworn by Hippocrates to heal the sick ought to exercise ferocity in the suppression of his inhalational urges lest he sow deadly nightshade in fertile minds. Nor do I have any patience at all with the addict who faces down his critics with a defiant *Fumo, ergo sum.* The reason why, dear reader, *I* continue against all reason to smoke is that I consider smoking a form of fumigation which is an ancient and venerable form of medical therapy, used by Paracelsus, among others, in the evacuation of demons from the possessed. It is precisely the warding off of demons with which I am concerned as I light a cigarette. Let those who would vilify me for this come forth with a better method of exorcism, and I promise I'll quit. Bunches of English rosemary were sold for six or eight pence on the street corners of London during the reign of Charles II in order to ward off the plague. Why, even the clergy, ever fastidious, carried little bouquets as they gave out Maundy money to the poor in Westminster Abbey. I know a sort of doctor who never makes a house call without a pomander of camphor and musk hidden in the gold head of his swagger stick—to ward off, I suppose, "ye foule stinkynge aire."

If anise or cinnamon were overrated as medicaments, it is equally true that a pledget of cotton soaked in oil of clove has numbed more than one aching tooth. And there is as yet no better way to coax urine from a recalcitrant postoperative female bladder than a sprinkling of oil of peppermint in the bedpan.

It is equally a blessing and a curse that the olfactory sense, like the sense of taste, is rapidly exhausted. I do think it somewhat unfair that the fatigued nose rids itself first of sweet odors, hanging on to stenches for what seems like ever, e.g. a dead mouse in the eaves. Although it is not so stated in *Hamlet*, one is confident that Gertrude lost no time in having Polonius hauled away from behind the arras in her bedchamber. The first sip of wine is the most exhilarating. Thereafter, the decline in acuity is steady until, with the final sip, one is so "full of the god" that he cannot smell anything at all. Thus, "good to the last drop" might be more properly, "OK to the dregs."

Likewise, it is the first inhalation of a rose that is strongest. The second is somewhat less. The third yet more pallid and so on until one might as well smell a frog as a flower. But switch from rose to hyacinth and the gates of Heaven swing open until, once again, the tired nose deadens itself to delight. Such nasal ennui is a blessing to those who work in hide-houses, tanneries, morgues, anatomy laboratories, or to those men who ply sanitation trucks.

As to the place of olfaction as it bears upon lust, there seems to be no set pattern. I for one have never smelled a pheromone such as the one Hero must have let fly across the Dardanelles to summon Leander. In this case, smell is a matter of taste. Some prefer their partners odorless and squeaky clean; others would plough a more alluvial plain. Aldonza the Whore was hardly an emblem of fastidity, yet enjoyed a reasonable popularity among the muleteers of rural Spain. Still, for the Man of La Mancha, Cervantes had her pasteurized to pure Dulcinea. Misguided efforts to control the spread of venereal disease have now and then involved the use of bad smells as anaphrodisiacs. The very logistics of impregnating the underwear of prostitutes with garlic or liederkranz leaves me faint; the damage this would do to the world of literature alone is staggering.

Were one to be robbed of any one of his senses, it were a lucky he who, retaining sight, sound, touch and taste, would give up his sense of smell. Still, like art which is necessary only in that without it life would be unbearable, smell is the sunset, the rainbow, the petal, the song. Live on after losing my smell? Like Bartleby the Scrivener, I prefer not to. A life is punctuated by smells without which it is an indecipherable message. Who could interpret the course of his life without the remembrance of horse manure, lilac, peony, lily of the valley, mothballs, wet dog, dead fish, pine woods, purple Concord grapes, Protestant churches opened Sunday morning after having been closed all week, certain Orthodox synagogues on Yom Kippur, the zeal of whose congregants is such as to prohibit even the brushing of their teeth. All of these inform me who I am, what I have done, what is the sum of my days. Familiar smells have an uncanny memory. One whiff of a childhood aroma can instantly recall bygone days. Thirty-five years ago, in the waiting room of his office, on the first floor of the house we lived in, my father was laid out for viewing. After the visitors and respects-payers had left, I stood alone in that room by the now closed casket. At its either end stood a tall floor lamp that gave off a red funerary light. The room was filled with a sweet, sickish smell which made me dizzy. It was with some effort that I tore myself at last from that scene of ultimate horror and ran upstairs. Three times since have I met that same smell, and each time, within the instant of recognition, the picture of my father in that room, those funerary lamps, the ruby gloom, all of it leaps untarnished into my mind's eye. Shelley knew this.

> *Odours when sweet violets sicken*
> *Live within the sense they quicken.*

And Bret Harte too:

> *The smell of that subtle sad perfume,*
> *As the spiced embalmings, they say, outlast*
> *The mummy laid in his rocky tomb,*
> *Awakes my buried past.*

Thus does the nose retrieve memories. It is the organ of nostalgia. O lilac! O new-mown hay! Only the most jaded of literary critics would lay aside unfinished a novel that begins: "The faint odor of Nuit de Noël perfume vividly recalls the Edgewater Beach Hotel in Chicago. It was August 1950. It was there I first met Florence—she was wearing this perfume. . . ." Immediately, we understand. It is we who remember Florence reeking with Nuit de Noël. And something else. Our prurient interest is aroused. We wonder. Whatever happened at the Edgewater Beach Hotel back in August 1950 between Florence and the narrator? Such speculation is the product of great art. On and on we read. Our pulse beats faster, saliva gathers in our mouth. We race to the elevator, up sixteen floors to room 1643. Inside, the room is dimly lit. A magnum of champagne rests in a bucket of ice . . . But I must not go on, Florence. It would be unfair to both of us.

Among the many utterances of Sigmund Freud with which one is free to take exception, is the pronouncement that *Riechlust*, the taking of libidinous pleasure in olfaction, is a mere phase, a childhood peccadillo that is consumed in the flames of puberty. Not so! A perfect sobersides of an electrical engineer confided in me that he was sexually aroused by grinding a handful of coffee beans, and inhaling the aroma. And I, myself, seldom fail to feel lascivious at the uncorking of a good Beaujolais.

Of the notions that have been misbestowed upon the nostrils, none is more spurious than that the size of the nose is directly correlated to the size of the penis. What seems applicable to elephants is simply not demonstrable in homo sapiens. The Romans, however, believed. It makes their chauvinistic attitude toward the "Roman nose" more understandable. All the germane jokes having been told and retold through the centuries, the myth of the nose *qua* penis has been quietly shelved. *Grace à Dieu*. This is not to suggest that the nose has no sexual application. It is not uncommon during sexual excitement for the nose to become stuffy and congested. The cause of this condition, known as "bride's nose," is unknown. But it is a plausible explanation for the run on Neo-Synephrine nasal spray during the month of June. What with amyl nitrite, Neo-Synephrine nose drops and birth control pills, one's honeymoon trousseau must include a portable medicine chest. A girl with a head on her shoulders would do well to search for a mate among the pharmacists of her village.

Be all that as it may, it is in the marriage of the tongue and the nose that taste is born. And here the nose is far the more discriminating. Versatile as it is in all other affairs, the tongue is rather a dull slug as a taster, being able to detect only the four gross tastes—sweet, sour, bitter, and salty. The delicate nose, on the other hand, discerns all the flavors of the world. That one can taste without having a tongue was demonstrated by the French surgeon LeCat, the same LeCat who gained fame by performing midthigh amputation on the battlefield in forty-five seconds. In 1750, LeCat tested two tongueless children, the one having been born without and the other having lost its tongue from smallpox. (Or so he claimed.) These two were quite able to distinguish among a wide variety of tastes. If further proof be needed, block up your nose and you will not know apple from potato. What child does not know to pinch his nose when taking medicine in order to kill the taste of it? One applauds the accuracy of the French who describe the "nose" of a wine. One deplores the carelessness of John Keats who "burst joy's grape against his palate fine." In the adult, there are no taste buds on the palate.

A person is born with ten thousand taste buds, each a little goblet-shaped cluster of cells one three-hundred-and-sixtieth of an inch across. In children, these buds are distributed widely over the tongue, the hard and soft palates, and the walls of the throat. By the time of puberty, only the tongue is so equipped. As you age, you lose your taste buds at a melancholy rate until, by the age of sixty, you have lost 65 percent of them. A thirteen-year-old will detect sweetness at one-third the concentration required by his grandfather. Therefore does the latter add more and more sugar and salt to his food. Those taste buds that survive lie at the tip, the sides, and the back part of the upper surface of the tongue. One experiences sweetness at the tip, saltiness at the sides and tip, sourness at the sides, and bitterness only at the back. Taste cells have a life span of only sixty days, constantly replenishing their number as the old ones disintegrate.

It is well known that man is not the only creature who tastes. The fly does it with his antennae; the sea anemone with his integument. Fish, newts, birds, and turtles taste. As does the mongoose who eats every bit of a rat except for the gall bladder whose bitter taste he cannot abide.

One god's nectar is another god's ipecac. One day, as writers will do, Goethe went calling on Schiller. Writers cleave unto one another much as the victims of a disease will form clubs whose meetings are designed not only for the dissemination of news, but for the tucking up of the spirits. For whatever reason—to gloat, to commiserate, to weep, to share a particularly vicious offense by his publisher, or to corroborate the hope that Schiller too was suffering from writer's block—Goethe visited Schiller. But it happened that Schiller was not at home. Perhaps he was calling on von Humboldt.

Whether aroused by the delicious temptation to snoop (a peek at Schiller's notebook; who could resist?), or else seized by some fierce inspiration of his own, Goethe sat himself down at Schiller's writing table until such time as the visitee should return. Almost at once, Goethe felt "a strange indisposition," a feeling of queasiness in the stomach which rose to the point of frank nausea and then to faintness. "A dreadful odor," Goethe recounts, "issued from a drawer near me. When I opened it I found, to my astonishment, that it was full of rotten apples." Pushing back the chair, Goethe staggered to the window of the room, flung it open, and leaned out. He inhaled deeply of the fresh air, and in a few minutes was revived.

Hearing the sounds of this activity, Schiller's wife entered the study, and, after hearing of Goethe's discomfort, explained that the drawer was always full of rotten apples, and that it was her wifely duty to keep it so. For, Frau Schiller further explained, the scent of rotten apples was beneficial to her husband. In fact, he could not write without it. As quickly as decorum would permit, Goethe departed from the premises, and it is doubtful that he ever again read a line of Schiller without feeling wamblings of nausea.

In the course of human events, rather more sophisticated use of the nose has been made. Maharanis have set their noses with rubies. There is a Filipino flute that is played with the nose. In the recesses of the nose, smugglers and spies have hidden secret messages, and witches poured vials of poison. Jealous caliphs have chained their concubines to nose rings. But it is as the organ of sexual expression that the nose has realized its highest purpose. It is no accident that the olfactory portion of the brain lies next to the center of the emotions. Nor is it without import that the olfactory lobes are called the testicles of the brain. Does not the swelling of a lusty nostril reveal the stallion's passionate intent?

For sheer beauty, consider only the philtrum, the sweet gully that, coursing as it does from the midline of the nose, participates in the shape of the lip. Here is a groove charmingly carved to admit the tip of the tongue, your own, or, with luck, someone else's. It follows that the cruelest fate has been visited upon the nose. It was ever thus. The greater the beauty of a thing, the more likely it is to suffer acts of madness. Worn at the very prow of the body, the nose is doubly vulnerable. It is true, is it not, that prey rushes forth to greet the hunter?

In India, for a thousand years, the usual and customary punishment for adultery was amputation of the nose, performed either by the injured party or by a designated *chuckler* stationed in the local bazaar. Nor was this unjust dessert served up for peccadillia only, but to discourage repetitive thievery as well. It was not uncommon for a conquering Indian army to commit metropolitan rhinocide, putting to the sword the nose of every man, woman, and child in the vanquished city. One supposes this done to prevent any revolutionary sniveling. And so it came to pass that the nation of India grew barren and nose poor. Nor was the sound of the sneeze to be heard in this land. At any time, in any place, were all the adulterers, thieves, and other losers to be so dismembered, the fully nosed person would become an endangered species. In the kingdom of the noseless, Pinocchio is king.

As luck would have it, there arose from among the Koomas, a certain small caste of Hindu bricklayers, a few men who were so distressed by the unkindness of these cuts that they set themselves the task of restoration of the nose. First, the edges of the nose stump were freshened by cutting away the scar. Next, a long, narrow pedicle of skin was raised from the forehead, leaving it attached narrowly between the eyes. This flap was then rotated, turned downward, and sutured to the stump of the nose. Just so the thing stood for some weeks like the handle of a pitcher until new blood vessels had bridged the gap between face and graft. Only then was the flap cut loose from the brow and, by a bit of judicious trimming and snippage, fashioned into a nose. The nostrils were held open by the insertion of metal tubes into the openings.

The Indian rhinoplasty was a huge success. Still, it was not until the sixteenth century that restoration of the nose was undertaken in Europe, the good nose doubtless having been brought from Bombay to Bologna by some itinerant surgeon or adulterer. Gaspare Tagliacozzi was professor of anatomy at the University of Bologna at a time when syphilis was epidemic in the European countries. Now, this disease blights, among other parts, the nose, chewing away the cartilage until the bridge collapses, and there is left but a hideous melted button that cannot be denied as the wages of sin. The sheepish owner of such a ruin takes on the smashed and abject look of the English bulldog.

Such were the gifts of Tagliacozzi that soon his clinic was crowded with soldiers, aristocratic ladies, cardinals, and princes. Tagliacozzi chose to use for his graft, not the forehead flap of Indian fame, but the flesh of the patient's upper arm. Three sides of a rectangle of tissue were elevated from the arm, and the free end stitched to the nose stump. Now the patient was encased in a metal and leather jacket which prevented the slightest movement. It was a device worthy of Nuremberg. Thus, face to armpit, the wretch remained for forty days and forty nights. This was followed by the separation and the final shaping. The patient was discharged from the clinic with the admonition not to take hold of his nose lest it part company with his face.

Brilliant were the results of this Italian Renasence. Unaccountably, the practice of restoration of the nose dwindled, possibly because of certain rumors that swirled through the salons and drawing rooms of the capitals of Europe. For one, it was bruited about that Tagliacozzi used the flesh of one man to construct the nose of another. One story, surely apocryphal, had it that the nose of a certain duke had formerly been part of the backside of a porter; still another, that the arm of a slave named Virax had been taken to make the nose of a Lord of Mantua, in return for which the slave had been granted manumission. Further, it was put abroad that the new nose was still subject to all the illnesses and accidents that were to befall its previous host, and that, should the freed slave, or whoever, die before the recipient, the new nose would blacken, shrivel, and fall off at that precise moment. Altogether a reprehensible distortion of history.

Even today, this calumny is advanced by irresponsible fictioneers in order to titillate their readers. As recently as 1974, one writer included such a tale, entitled "The Sympathetic Nose," in a collection of short stories. The name of this vain scamp I choose not to mention lest he fail to sink into the oblivion that he so richly deserves. Suffice it to say that for three centuries the operation of restoration of the nose languished in disuse until its revival in nineteenth century England.

All of which brings us to that peculiar phenomenon of cosmetic surgery—rhinoplasty—for the practice of which a whole guild of nose mongers was formed. One wonders whether the idea of cosmetic rhinoplasty is not a throwback to another operation performed by the ancient surgeons, *decoris causa*, that being the surgical lengthening of a preternaturally short foreskin so that it would cover the glans penis. Of this latter procedure, the surgeon Fabricius ab Aquapendente has this to say, "Any great desire to render these parts more attractive seems somewhat superfluous." (Free translation.)

What, then, is one to say about the advent of mass rhinoplasty? True, it is most cleverly done, the scars artfully concealed, the risks, although present, relatively minor, the discomfort well within the bounds of the notion that one must suffer for his beauty. Still, is there something not a little sad in a philosophy which insists that a bit less nose can make you happy? If joy depends upon the excision of one half-ounce of nose, then did the capacity for joy ever exist? Is it less than arrogance to set standards of beauty that are other than Nature's own? Besides, in our very variety is our beauty.

Consider the prospect of a planet full of identical noses,

each one pert, narrow, a bit retroussé, and modeled after some ideal of beauty that may well be no more than a commercialized fad limited to his country, and which future generations may group with the bound feet of eighteenth century China and the castrated boys of the old Middle East. Such a sameness would give us little cause to take notice of each other. In buying these anonymous plastic noses, we risk losing yet another taste, that for the subtle and infinite differences that make us dear to one another.

Surgeons, wouldst arm the Venus de Milo? Head the Winged Victory of Samothrace? Breathes there a sculptor so craven, so callow that he would mix sand and water to fashion a nose for the Sphinx? A pug, say? Or a bulbous? Such a man does not know that life is a succession of missing fragments. No, the truth is that there is no stone which holds imprisoned the as yet uncarved replacement for the Sphinx's nose. Let the Sphinx be! He is incompleteness mutely verified, yet undeniably the better for it.

And so ye potato-, pug-, hog-, shovel-, parrot-, hawk-, and dog-nosed folk, all ye who, disappointed in your physiognomy, yearn for rhinoplasty, take care that in cutting off your ancestral nose, ye do not spite your soul. If you are Cyrano, then, by God, *be* Cyrano, and deal with Fate accordingly. There is dignity in such an uneven struggle, and more beauty than in ten thousand anatomical lies.

THE HARTFORD GIRL

ON A FRIDAY night in August 1976, in the city of Hartford, something happened. The newspaper reported it like this:

A sixteen-year-old girl slashed her wrists and arms and then rushed to the steps of a Roman Catholic church poking a razor to her throat while a crowd of three hundred persons cheered and screamed, "Do your thing, sister!" For forty-five minutes she held back police and priests by threatening to cut her throat. Finally she collapsed on the steps of Immaculate Conception Church because she lost so much blood. Three bottles were thrown by the crowd which hooted as the girl staggered on the steps of the church. One bottle struck the girl and the others smashed against the church and the street curb. While the girl bled profusely, one man jumped up on the sidewalk and recited a brief couplet of doggerel verse. Three more times she cut her arms with the razor and each time the crowd applauded. A cheer rose from the mob when the girl finally fainted and collapsed from loss of blood. Police took her to the hospital. A dozen persons went to look at the pools of blood that had dripped from the girl's arms after she was taken away.

That is what the newspaper reported. Nor is it to be challenged. Doubtless, it is all true, all correct. But sitting here at a desk, with a pencil in my hand, the event takes on a reality more intense than that which is said to have happened in Hartford that night. Just so does wakefulness or myth reveal our changeless ancestral themes . . .

It is ten-thirty at night.

The girl's name is Catherine. I heard someone say that. She has long black hair. She is barefoot, and is wearing a sleeveless white shirt and dungarees that have been cut off at the knee. The unstitched edges are raveled.

Some said it was the heat that made her do it. Others said she had taken drugs—LSD or speed. But I don't know. It might as well have been the moon, some wild wind blowing, a shifting of chemicals at the base of her brain, the way ice cracks at one place on a river, no one knows why, and after that the smooth white spread is buckled in that place.

No one saw where she came from. All at once, she was there on the street corner, and in her hand, a razor that she raised and brought down across her wrist and arm. She was no expert. That was plain to see. She had to swipe again and again, biting her lower lip with her teeth until at last she made it to an artery. Already the crowd was gathering. How quickly it materialized! As though summoned from beneath the pavement to enact with her here. Soon her blood was answered by a smattering of applause. "Right on, sister!" There is laughter. Another shout, "Do your thing!" As if to show that laughter is power, the razor, like an acrobat, turned boisterous, and leaped to her other hand, flicking blood from the second wrist. Or did the loyal blood chase the blade from the small new wound it had made?

The crowd had grown to about three hundred. A circle has formed about the girl, hemming her in. I am standing on the stoop of a house across the street. I am here . . .

because . . . I belong here. Now the girl raises the point of the razor to her throat, holds it rigid, emphatic, over the exact place where I know the jugular vein and the carotid artery course alongside the trachea. How does she know this anatomy? She backs slowly toward the ring of people. At first the circle holds, then abruptly shudders and breaks to let her through, the way a single bush in a field will shake until the branches part in one place, and a sparrow is disgorged. In any case, the circle parts. No one wants to be soiled by the blood. She could be dangerous!

Free once more, she breaks into a kind of crouching run. The crowd follows, hawking her. Once she stumbles, drops to one knee, but it is momentary. She rises running. Now her movements are full of grace, all tiptoe equipoise, now she is awkward, jerking herself along the pavement like a lizard through tall grass. In the middle of the block looms a church. The Church of the Immaculate Conception! Broad stone steps lead up from the street to the great wooden doors, shut and locked for the night. Above the arched doorway, twin censing angels hold braziers aloft. She mounts the steps, then turns to face the people of Hartford. The razor waits at her neck. No one climbs the steps.

The first bottle is hurled.

It smashes on the steps just below her. Shards fly up toward her dazzled feet. Points of blood appear. They trail down toward her toes. She seems puzzled, weary. She drops her arms. There is the noise of a bolt being drawn behind her, and the massive church door opens. A priest appears in the doorway. He takes one step toward the girl, then stops. She has seen him and once again raises the blade to her neck. He dare not come closer.

There is more laughter. Someone cheers. A comic man at the front of the crowd jumps up to the lowest step, whips around, and recites a couplet of verse in a high singsong voice, then leaps back to his place. Loud applause. Far away a siren sounds. The girl cocks her head to listen. Her body grows tense as the siren approaches. She will not be taken by surprise. Two policemen arrive. "Move along," they command those nearest them. They shove and shoulder to the forefront. But never do they ascend to her place.

The second bottle catches her in the side and falls unbroken to the steps. She buckles, then straightens.

"Stop that!" shouts the priest.

"Who threw that bottle?" cries a policeman.

Now the girl is wild and pale. Like the bride of Lammermoor. She raises her unarmed arm from which the clots loop, and stretches out her black hair behind her, taut as the strings of a cello, then lets it fall. From the door of the church, a faint odor of incense wafts across the street.

She is weakening. I can see it in the tremor that seizes her upraised arm. It spreads, becomes a wobbling that causes her whole body to wave like poured cream. The third bottle strikes the front of the church just behind her. She does not hear it, for just then, very slowly, she billows down the stone steps to fall among her clots. She is like the white center of a huge red-petaled flower, a peony. Now the crowd is hushed. Look! She moves one final time, then lies still. The bells of the church are as quiet as blood.

The priest and the police are bending over her. Tourniquets are applied. She is carried to an ambulance and taken away.

Almost at once, the crowd begins to dissipate. The people seem strangely spent, melancholy. A woman crosses herself, and climbs the church steps to stand near the blood. She is joined by others. They bend to examine it closely, murmuring. For a moment, I wonder if they are going to kneel and lap this blood from the church steps. But now they, too, leave, and the street is empty.

It is months later. Still, whenever I think of beauty, I think of her.

THE LAMMERGEIER

I AM ALONE and trekking the sterile desert of Sinai. Is it a quest that I have undertaken? No, it is more a hunt, with all that suggests of blood and combat. But I do not know the nature of my quarry. I know only that it is here among these rifts and escarpments that I shall find him.

It is hot. With each breath, the desiccated air scrapes my lungs. Here in the Sinai, the legend of the Burning Bush is plausible. There is no single tree to console the tangled ridges tossed up blood red against the sky. Only sandstone cliffs and mounds of granite sculpted by the wind. This is no torrid climate, but a fever of the land.

I am standing on a ledge near the top of a rocky slope. Below is a valley that is hardly more than a broad ravine. Across this declivity is another barren rise. It is identical to the one upon which I stand. Perhaps it is the same one. I cannot be certain of anything here. In the heat, my eyes are melting. All at once I see, motionless upon a narrow ledge near the top of the hill opposite me, a white ram. His body seems painted upon the rock face, like a drawing on the wall of a cave. His head presents above the summit, so that his braided horns silhouette against the sky. Upon what does he feed? What drink? Here, where there is neither leaf nor dew? He seems to me pure, immaculate, a forgotten god, perhaps, reappearing in the guise of a ram to inhale once again the ancient odor of sacrifice.

In the Sinai, time is not the steady progression of years and events, but is as often the past recapitulated. So it is that I see in the distance a vast plain from which a plume of blue smoke is sucked upward and laid against the sky. I follow the column of smoke to its source, and I see another white ram. The legs of this ram are bound, and the animal lies upon its side. Two men dressed in the skins of beasts lift the ram to a stone altar. One of the men grasps the horns of the ram and bends the head backward to present the throat. I hear chanting. There is the flash of a blade, a sudden bib of blood upon the white fleece. A third man appears. He raises the horn of a ram to his lips. One of his hands holds the narrow stem, the other cradles the flare. The head of the priest tilts backward. And echoing across the Sinai comes that sound that is the groan and sputter of the heart torn open and gushing prayer. Now the scene is enveloped in flames. Soon there is only that plume of blue smoke sucked upward and rubbing against the sky.

I turn to gaze across the ravine. Behold the ram! The twists of whose fleece are like unto the curled surface of the brain. How solemn and changeless his countenance. He is suspended above the burnt-out desert in a state of utter passiveness and indifference. High above, a speck hangs in the sky. It vanishes, then draws nearer, circling. I know at once that it is he for whom I have been searching. It is the lammergeier. Huge, he rides the thermal updrafts from the Sinai, idling, reddening himself on the sun. In a moment, there is a noise of blankets flapping, and the great bird stoops to the ram on the ledge. His talons catch the fire of the sun. His beak, too, ignites. His very neck is bearded with flame. The ram, in stillness, waits.

At a hundred miles an hour, the lammergeier hammers the ram. The fire of the bird spreads to the ram. It arcs between his horns as he tumbles down the steep slope into the valley, where he lies as still in death as he was in life. As though the fact of his life or death were incidental to his stillness. To a god, what does it matter?

As swiftly as he had come, the lammergeier is gone. Hours go by; the shadows of the hills encroach upon the ravine where the white ram lies bloating. I descend into the valley. Once again, there is a rushing sound, and now I see the lammergeier embedded upon the weltering carcass, mantling it with his wings. From the rear, he is like a surgeon bending over an open abdomen. His head dives, pulls. I move closer. Something draws me.

The floor of the ravine is strewn with splintered bones. I recognize the distal half of a femur, the broken skull of an ibex. Ahead, a large flat rock, perhaps twenty feet on each side, glares from the dusty floor of the ravine. Here, the bony fragments are more numerous. The surface of the rock is stained darkly. Blood? Excrement? All the while, unmindful of my presence, the lammergeier feeds upon the ram. It is growing darker. A white moon appears in the sky. In the pallor, the ram begins to lose its clarity, graying out first at the periphery, then everywhere. Even as the ram dissolves, the lammergeier grows more distinct, more real, so that each groove and feather stands apart from its neighbor. A moment later there is the sound of wings, and the lammergeier is once again aloft. In his talons, he carries the thighbone of the ram. Quickly, he ascends to a great height above the Sinai. Then, hurtles across the ravine. From two hundred feet above, he lets loose the bone. With a desolate clatter, it strikes the rock that is the ossuary of the lammergeier. Braking, the bombardier turns in his own hot wind, and dips to the place where the shattered bone lies. And I, so close I can see him beaking his twice-slain work, see his long scooped tongue probing the hollow shaft for the marrow.

I know now that I have come here to die. This is the

secret I have been waiting to be told. The lammergeier is looming. I shall be his prey, buffeted by him. Through the dusk, I peer at the vague pale crumple that was the ram. It is *myself* that I see. A wind rises, disturbing only the skin, the hair, the globes of my eyes. The Sinai, which had been as silent as bone, is now filled with sound. It is a long undisciplined moan that I have known all my life. It is the sound of the ram's horn. The noise terrifies me, and I wheel about to find its source. At first, it seems to emerge from a cloud, but then I see that there is a tall cleft rock adjacent to the flat rock that is the ossuary of the lammergeier. It is this cleft rock which, when struck by the wind, emits the notes I hear. I am trembling. I strain to hear above the dreadful music the rushing of his wings. When will he strike?

In a state of madness, I fall to the ground, waiting. But he does not come. For a long time, I lie there holding myself rigid for the impact that I know is coming. But the lammergeier does not come. It is toward dawn. The wind has gone and with it the sound of the ram's horn. With the gathering light, my fear lessens. I grow crafty. *I will not die.* Not this day. More than ever, I feel surging the instinct of my tissues to remain alive. But I must prepare. A plan forms in my brain. It is so audacious that, for a moment, I have an impulse to laugh. As the sun appears in the sky, I mount to the platform of the ossuary. I open my shirt and take the knife from my belt. Islanded among skulls, I lie upon my back. Four quick strokes with the point of the knife bring blood screening across my chest. I toss the knife from me, and I lie spread-eagle upon the rock. Minute by minute, the heat rises. My skin is scorching. I grow dizzy, faint.

I feel myself to be profoundly ill in some way. As though something, a tumor, were growing inside me. It is this tumor that is the favorite meat of the lammergeier. And it is only he that can extirpate it from my body. With his beak, his talons. I close my eyes. Perhaps I sleep. Perhaps I lie upon an operating table; a surgeon bends above me; his scalpel flashes.

When I open my eyes, I see, as through a gauze of heat, the lammergeier crowding. His beak, only inches from my breast. But I am no white ram! My human hands shoot up, the one to capture his legs just above the awful claws, the other to seize his neck. And we are engaged! Again and again, he batters me with his outspread wings; then, heaving upward, he strains to regain the air. He would fly. But he cannot. I am too heavy a weight to be taken from the earth. And I will not let him go.

Just so, all day, do I hold against the wild beating of his wings. Just so do I remain, arched and taut, squeezing until the bird hangs limp between my fists. At last, unbolting, I drop what is now no more than a bundle of snapped twigs. And I awaken to exhaustion.

But a pain has crossed from dream to wakefulness, and I feel it in the hollow of my thigh. Rising to one elbow, I examine the dark bruise where the lammergeier has struck me.

Twice, I have dreamt of the lammergeier. I carry him in my blood. A man can deny that his death approaches, busy himself with labor and pleasure. But what can he do with his dreams? Those honest messengers. Oh, I shall dream of the lammergeier again. I shall have another turn with him. The pain in my thigh that has pursued me, it binds me to him. It is a covenant between us. There will be his fiery plumage, his arrowy stoop. The hit! Perhaps the next time he will kill me. Perhaps he will cut out of my belly the tumor that he loves. And I shall feel his marrow-scooping tongue deep. Ah, deep! Lick deeper! Inside my bones.

APPENDIX

And I said to him, "Dicky Bird, why do you cry
    Willow, Tit Willow, Tit Willow?
Is it absence of intellect, Birdy?" I cried.
"Or a rather tough worm in your little inside?"
With a shake of his poor little head he replied,
    "Willow, Tit Willow, Tit Willow."

Koko's Song, The Mikado

JUST SUPPOSE that you have in your ownership one of those elongated balloons whose walls, rather than being smooth, are haustrated into incomplete segments, like links of knockwurst. And suppose that you have been asked by a child to blow up the balloon. Agreeably, you begin, puffing mightily and watching with partially crossed eyes as the pretty thing expands. It is very satisfying. The child waits at your knee, his great dark eyes enkindled with awe. And so it goes. But midway in the enterprise, something is amiss. A sudden uphill tendency is realized. You are having trouble. You shift into a lower gear; it does no good. Soon, as much air leaks out as you are able to stuff in. The child waits at your knee, his great dark eyes now fixed (with what you see as sangfroid) upon the engorged veins of your neck,

217

the sweat that breaks upon your brow, the plethoric red of your face. That you are in imminent danger of bursting something other than the balloon is news that the child does not want to hear. Only the report Done! There you are! will send him on his way.

Madly now, you chew the damp little nozzle, biting it to stop the outrush of precious air. With mounting panic, you gather for the next blast. And all at once, you have no blast to gather; no, nor any hollow hiss. Only the loose wet thudding that tells of yet another bit of ground lost.

Now, no man of decent family connection suffers gladly a humiliation before the eyes of his child. Such ignominy will come your way without galloping toward it. All too soon, one's progeny discover that their father (good grief!) has touched the dark underside of life, or that he cannot Indian-wrestle them to the floor without a furtive lapse of the foot rules. Or that he cannot blow up all the way a mere sausage balloon.

But to the business! At last, you can do no more. One more huff and you will throw up, you will faint. Green-gold spots explode in your eyes. You pinch off the cervical stump of the balloon, and you twist it into a knot. You hand the balloon to the child. "There," you gasp.

"You didn't get it all the way up," he says. "It's not all the way up." You have heard these words before, in another time, another place. You have seen such expressions on other faces. No longer do you give a fig for the child's dark-eyed awe. You are far too dizzy for adoration. A familiar feeling steals over you. It is a strange blend of self-loathing and infanticide.

That the child is correct in his perceptions is undeniable. No amount of guile will deflect his attention from the fact that at the farther end of the balloon, there remains a fingerling, an udderlet, that is uninflated as the day it was manufactured. There it hangs like a proclamation of impotence. Something else has faded here besides your own resources; it is the child's certainty that you can do anything, that you are strong as a Viking, and six times as amusing. Not without some regret, you watch his dream fade. Ah, let it go. Let it go.

Certain soulless endeavors do not allow for dissembling. Balloon blowing is one of them. You simply cannot pretend to a child that a balloon is fully inflated when it has that little thing hanging at the end. If only balloon blowing did not demand perfection. If only it were customary to accept something less than the absolute, then one could be graded on a sliding scale. In which case, a compassionate child could be trained to cry out, when the final three inches remain undistended, "Bravo! You got 85%!" and rush off proudly to send the airy fraction soaring.

Where is all this leading? To the appendix, of course. Let us go then, you and I, to retrieve from that ungrateful child the sausage balloon. Now stand before a long mirror and hold the balloon in front of your midsection such that the balloon is bent into an inverted U, the nozzle being placed low down on the left, and the unfilled nubbin somewhat less far down on your right. Notice how the terminal three inches of recent shame projects from the full-blown corpus of the thing. Now, if the great swollen air-filled part is your colon, and the nozzle is your anus, then your appendix is that professor of humility that presides over your right lower abdomen.

With what could the Great Shaper have been preoccupied when he so miscalculated the intestinal length necessary for the treatment of the aliments of man? Could he have been so enthralled with his work on the helix of the ear? Was it some lingering indecision over the fingers? To web or not to web? Surely it was no Divine malice that brought man to his misgutment. Whatever, there it hangs, a misplaced comma in an otherwise sensible essay. Having no function and capable of none, it is not even a spare part. It is but an accessory. And given, O deviltry, the shape of a worm!

Other parts are expendable, the gall bladder, the spleen, the odd digit or tonsil, but none of these is so lacking in purpose as to be of no earthly use to the community of organs. No so the appendix. If proof were needed that the pig is at least as well set up as man, the more capacious appendix of the pig does take part in the digestive process. Is it not ironic that the one part of the corpus most useless, most lacking in anatomical and physiological importance should be the one part most commonly diseased? The appendix is the evil dwarf who will cut any caper in order to get attention. Give ear:

At some point in its narrow canal, the appendix becomes obstructed. A vagrant pebble of inspissated stool, perhaps, is pushed by peristalsis into the neck of the appendix. Further contractions shove the "fecalith" deeper into the blind alley. At last it stops, impacted. Like a fat chimney sweep that finds himself stuck *in medias res*, the pebble cannot be dislodged. There it sits, accruing unto itself more and more of the effluent, which stuff is packed about the nidus of the thing so that it grows larger and larger, presses ever more insistently against the lining of the appendix. Too late: The worm understands that it has bitten off more than it can chew. The little veins at the site of compression are occluded; they can no longer lead away the blood that has been delivered by the arteries.

The appendix becomes engorged; it swells, impaling itself further against the fecal stone that it harbors. The arteries are next to be shut off, and with that, the blood supply to the appendix ceases. The appendix begins to die.

First, the mucosal lining ulcerates; next, the muscular layer is overrun; the usually harmless bacteria that inhabit the colon turn mean and invade the necrotic tissues. At last, the third, the final layer, the serosa, is invaded. The appendix has gone from pink to purple to green and then to black in the rainbow of gangrene. A tiny increment in pressure and . . . perforation! Out bursts the fecalith into the abdominal cavity, rolling, tumbling, sliding between the shocked loops of bowel to bounce into the lateral gutters of the belly and down into the pelvis, where it festers alongside the innocent ovary, the fallopian tube. Through the ragged rupture runs a river of pus and stool, soiling, inflaming, scalding, setting fire to the peritoneum wherever it puddles.

Not by stool alone, however, has the worm been turned. Such oddments and endments as nails, tacks, screws, pits, kernels of corn, and the seeds of innumerable fruits and vegetables may act with equal villainy. I, myself, have cut into the freshly removed appendix of a succotash addict to find there, flourishing sweetly in darkness and manure, a germinating lima bean with well-developed cotyledons.

And so . . . peritonitis. Now fever burns; there is nausea and vomiting; the slightest motion of your body ruffles the stagnant lake within and brings on new rhapsodies of pain. Left to your fate, you would surely become a matter of interest to your clergyman and your heirs. Only the knife can save you now, and that blade from which in better days you would have shrunk in horror, you now embrace with ardor. Lickety-split, the ruptured appendix is removed, and its fecal escapee recaptured. The grateful peritoneum cleans up the rest of the mess. In time, all that will remain upon the plain of battle will be a few fine adhesions.

It is the tradition that young surgeons in training cut their teeth on appendectomies, these baptismal operations done under the direct guidance of experienced older men. As a teacher of surgery, I have played Vergil to countless Dantes on their initial descent into Hell. So many of these young surgeons and medical students have fainted during the operation of appendectomy that I have begun to suspect that there is some hitherto undetected toxic flatus released by the uncovered appendix that lays these youthful aspirants green and sweating on the operating room floor. Against these fumes, we elder sawbones have developed the immunity of repeated exposure, and, luckily, are able to complete the operation so interrupted. By just such serendipity have many of the great medical truths been discovered.

A few intrepid men have removed their own appendices. Some, because there was no one else around to do it; others, because it was there. Despite its obvious appeal to the professional acrobat, the merely double-jointed amateur, and the devotee of unusual sex practices, autoappendectomy remains a rare phenomenon upon which students of behavior need dwell no further.

It is true, is it not, that literature reflects life? While certain species of worm chew through a book, chapter and verse, sparing not metaphor, not cliché; it is, ultimately, the appendix that finishes things off.

Apres lui, rien!

ABOUT THE AUTHOR

RICHARD SELZER is a native of Troy, New York. Born in 1928, the son of a general practitioner, he was educated at Union College, Albany Medical College, and Yale. He has been in the practice of general surgery since 1960 in New Haven, Connecticut, and is on the faculty of the Yale School of Medicine.

A collection of Richard Selzer's short stories entitled *Rituals of Surgery* was published in 1974. In 1975, he won the National Magazine Award for his essays. *Mortal Lessons*, a book of essays, was published in 1976.

He lives with his wife and three children in New Haven.